Published in 2005 by:
Nelson Thornes Ltd
Delta Place
27 Bath Road
CHELTENHAM
GL53 7TH
United Kingdom

05 06 07 08 09 / 10 9 8 7 6 5 4 3 2 1

A catalogue record for this book is available from the British Library

ISBN 0 7487 8584 1

Illustrations by Peters & Zabransky Ltd
Page make-up by Northern Phototypesetting Co. Ltd, Bolton

Printed in Great Britain by Scotprint

Contents

Acknowledgements

The author and publishers are grateful to the following for permission to reproduce copyright material in this tutor support pack:

- Crown copyright/MOD material is reproduced with the permission of the Controller of Her Majesty's Stationery Office © Crown copyright. All rights reserved. Core click-use licence no.C02W0002214

Every attempt has been made to contact copyright holders, and we apologise if any have been overlooked. Should copyright have been unwittingly infringed in this book, the owners should contact the publishers, who will make corrections at reprint.

Grateful thanks to Wayne Thorne, Carole Buckley and Eric Buckley for their continual support and encouragement.

Special thanks to my colleagues at Hastings College: Keith Leech, Anthony Powell, Maria Lehane, Sally Richardson, Heather Grief and Penny McLean.

Dedicated as always with love and thanks to my wonderful daughters Alexandria and Natasha.

Introduction

For many Access students, human anatomy and physiology will be their first in-depth study of a biological science. This subject provides an insight into how the body is structured and the mechanisms of body functions and the implications for healthcare.

Anatomy and physiology begins with a single cell called a zygote and this develops into the unique and complex multi-cellular structure of the human body. Anatomists have been studying the human body for centuries. Egyptian artefacts prove that ancient civilisations used knowledge of anatomy for medicinal and religious practice. In the London Science Museum, some of the Roman surgical and dissecting instruments that are displayed are very similar to the instruments used today.

Modern technology has enabled the subject of human anatomy and physiology to be explored in great detail, but due to the complexity of the body many questions still remain unanswered.

The difference between anatomy and physiology

When studying the human body it is important to understand the difference between anatomy and physiology.

Anatomy relates to the structure of the human body and includes all organs from cell structure to groups of tissues that have specific shape and form.

Physiology relates to how the structures of the human body work and function.

To gain a full understanding of how the body functions it is necessary to incorporate several other branches of science including:

- Chemistry: to gain insight into the composition of matter and reactions between different types of matter.

- Physics: to understand the behaviour and characteristics of matter. Matter is the term used for anything that occupies a space. In anatomy and physiology a space is usually an area that contains a fluid or gas. A potential space implies that matter (for example air or blood) may enter that space if ill health occurs.

- Sociology: to explore how social behaviour affects the health and well-being of individuals.

- Psychology: to understand the links between perceptions of health and illness.

The relationship between anatomy and physiology is delicately balanced to allow the body to work effectively and efficiently to ensure survival. Homeostasis is the name given to the process which maintains the stability of the body and ensures that the needs of all the cells are being met in order that they can function. This is an automatic and self-regulating process which is necessary for health and well-being.

Homeostasis is dependent upon the internal and external environments. The internal environment refers to mechanisms that regulate body function and essential chemical processes that regulate the internal consistency of body fluids surrounding the cells. The external environment relates to the conditions we live in and includes factors such as temperature, air quality, altitude and social settings.

A holistic approach to care requires an understanding of the biological, sociological and psychological aspects of health. Healthcare professionals have a duty of care to their clients and part of this duty includes an understanding of anatomy and physiology. In order to effectively meet the needs of individual clients, knowledge of the functions of the human body is essential when planning care. The outcome of care may be predicted with greater accuracy when there is knowledge of the process of homeostasis.

Before clients can be autonomous in making decisions about healthcare, they will need guidance in order to make an informed choice. Healthcare professions must therefore be able to advise clients in detail of how best to maintain health and the implications of behaviour that fails to provide an environment promotes homeostasis.

An understanding of how the body functions will assist in the health worker's role as an observer. Recordings of measurements of body functions such as blood pressure, pulse and temperature need to be compared with normal–range values and knowledge is required of the importance and consequences of any variations observed.

Normal structure and function of the human body is essential for homeostasis. If there is a breakdown in any of the systems of the human body, illness or health deficiencies may ensue.

Structure of the book

The human body is a complex and amazing structure. This book is aimed at providing Access students with a basic knowledge of human biology and an introduction to the terminology used to describe the many different aspects of anatomy and physiology.

To assist students as they progress to further studies in human biology the terms used in this book are common to all anatomy and physiology texts. For example, diagrams use anatomical terms to describe which section of an organ is being viewed. The body may be divided into three different planes so that the reader can understand the position and location of the different body structures.

Planes – imaginary lines that divide the body

Proximal end of upper limb

Distal end of upper limb

Posterior (dorsal)

Anterior (ventral)

Dorsal surface of hand

Palmar surface of hand

Superior

Inferior

(a) Median plane   **(b) Transverse plane**   **(c) Coronal plane**

a. Median or mid-sagittal plane: divides an organ in half.

b. Transverse plane: divides into upper and lower sections.

c. Coronal or frontal plane: divides into front and back sections.

To help you with your studies this book has been set out in chapters that divide the body into different systems, as follows:

- Cells and tissues.

- The skeleton and movement: the bony structures needed for support and movement.

- Cardiovascular system: heart, blood vessels and blood.

- The nervous and endocrine systems: the brain and nerves.

- Respiratory system: the lungs.

- Digestive system: supplying nutrients to all cells.

- Genital-urinary system: kidneys and the reproductive system.

- Defence systems: including special senses of sight, hearing, taste, touch and smell.

- Stress and illness: the relationship between psychology and physiology.

- Disease and disorders: causes of ill health.

Each chapter sets out learning outcomes that will be achieved after study and may be useful as a study guide when revising for written tests. Diagrams that you may be required to draw during tests have been produced for you to copy. These are indicated at the beginning of each chapter and are also marked with a *. With so many different systems and organs to learn you may find it helpful to colour in the diagrams, using the colour keys (you will need a set of 24 colouring pencils). This may help you to revise and it will be a welcome change from simply reading the text. Although the chapters examine different systems of the body, you should remember that all systems work together to maintain homeostasis. Therefore, each chapter contains information on how that system affects other systems in the body.

There may be many words with which you are unfamiliar. To help you with pronunciation of the more difficult names, the phonetic spellings are included in brackets. It is important to learn how to pronounce words correctly so that you can familiarise yourself with terminology commonly used in a work-based setting. In the phonetic spellings capital letters are used to show where emphasis is placed. Some words are quite long and often have two places of emphasis. Strong emphasis on letters is shown by ' and unstressed letters are not marked. A medical dictionary may prove helpful in your studies.

Details of diseases and disorders are included at the end of each chapter. The conditions are described briefly and there are a few examples of the different types of disorders that occur in the various systems. There is a list of further reading at the end of each chapter and this may be useful if you are required to present an in-depth study of specific diseases and disorders.

Reading the relevant chapters before your lectures will help you to gain an insight and understanding of the subject matter. During your lessons you may have the opportunity to examine anatomical structures and participate in laboratory dissection. The use of anatomical models and dissection is an excellent learning tool and very useful for consolidating your knowledge of the structure of body organs.

Chapter 1
Cells and tissues

National unit specification
These are the topics you will be studying for this unit.

1   Cells

2   Tissues

3   Homeostasis

Diagram to practise:
Structure of a cell

1 Cells

Cytology is the study of cells. Information gained on the structure and function of individual cells will give a greater understanding of disease and disorders that affect the human body.

Our bodies are made up of cells that develop from a single cell called the zygote, a fertilised human egg. The cell develops into groups of specialised cells.

Each zygote contains deoxyribonucleic acid (DNA) which carries the genetic blue-print for the structure and function of all cells. The human body is a multicellular organism containing billions of different cells that each have a specific function.

The function of all organs is based on the anatomical and chemical structure of the specialised cells. Every organ in the body has a direct or indirect relation-ship with other organs to create and maintain an environment of physical and chemical harmony called homeostasis (hō′mē-ō′STĀ-sis), which is necessary for function and survival.

Human cell structure

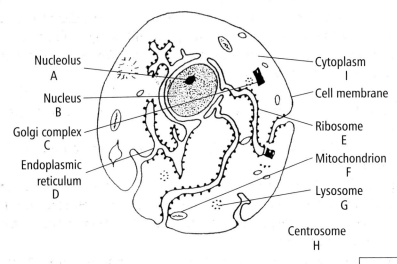

Nucleolus
A

Nucleus
B

Golgi complex
C

Endoplasmic
reticulum
D

Cytoplasm
I

Cell membrane

Ribosome
E

Mitochondrion
F

Lysosome
G

Centrosome
H

* Diagram to practise

A	=	Green
B	=	Orange
C	=	Brown
D	=	Light blue
E	=	pink
F	=	Red
G	=	Dark blue
H	=	Purple
I	=	Yellow

The three parts of a cell

Each cell in the human body contains similar internal components.

- **Cell membrane** (plasma membrane): a very fine membrane that allows substances to pass in and out across the membrane, to nourish and remove waste products from the cell, by means of:
    - Diffusion: substances from a higher concentration on one side of the membrane pass through to a lower concentration until the substances on both sides of the membrane have equal concentration. Only small molecules are able to pass through in this way.
    - Osmosis: water passes through the membrane from a weaker to a stronger concentration until solutions on both sides are equal.
    - Facilitated osmosis: molecules become attached to a carrier molecule called a lysosome, and are transported through the membrane. Facilitated osmosis occurs when substances that are too large to diffuse need to be carried across and released on the other side.
    - Active transport: substances transfer through the membrane regardless of their concentration by the use of energy from within the cell in the form of adenosine triphosphate (ah-DEN-ō-sēn tri-FOS-făt) (ATP).
    - Phagocytosis and pinocytosis: the membrane may engulf particles or substances. Once inside the cell the particles are broken down by chemical reactions and ingested by the cytoplasm. (An example of this is the action of white cells ingesting bacteria.)
- **Cytoplasm:** the protoplasm that is inside the cell around the nucleus. Protoplasm is a jelly-like substance containing the following molecules:
    - Organelles: structures that have specific functions. There are different types of organelles, each one has a different enzyme.
    - Endoplasmic reticulum (en'-dō-PLAS-mik re-TIK-yoo-lum): a network of membranes that form sacs called cisterns. The outer surface contains ribosomes.
    - Ribosomes contain ribonucleic acids (RNA): these join amino acids into protein chains.
    - The golgi complex is made up of molecules that process the protein chains and deliver to parts of the cell requiring chemical input. Lysosomes originate in the golgi complex which are capable of breaking down chemical components of the cell.
    - Mitochondria: the energy source of the cell. Nutrients are burnt using oxygen to produce energy. The energy is stored in the molecular carrier, adenosine triphosphate (ATP).
    - Vacuoles: clear spaces which may contain waste material.

- **Nucleus:** a central mass containing nucleoplasm surrounded by a nuclear membrane. It maintains intercellular homeostasis.
    - Near the nucleus is a round body called the centrosome that contains two small circular bodies called the centrioles.
    - The nucleus stores the genetic material DNA.
    - RNA is required to transfer the information from the DNA to the ribosomes that produce proteins.

Endoplasmic reticulum and ribosomes

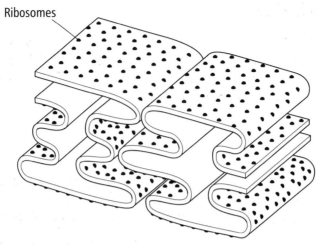

Division of cells (mitosis)

Individual cells multiply by cell division. The shape of the cell will depend upon its function, which is determined by the nuclei of the cell that contains the genes. The genes are the DNA molecules and DNA must be duplicated during cell division.

The process of mitosis

- Prophase: the centrosome divides and remains connected by thread-like strands. The chromatin becomes more defined and forms 23 pairs of rod-like structures called chromosomes and these contain DNA. Each chromosome divides into two, attached to the centre point of the thread-like strands.

- Metaphase: the nuclear membrane disappears and the centrosomes go to opposite poles of the cell with the chromosomes attached to the centomere in the middle.

- Anaphase: the centomere divides and the two identical chromosomes move apart, breaking the thread-like strands.

- Telophase: the cell constricts around the middle and a nuclear membrane forms. The cell divides forming two identical daughter cells.

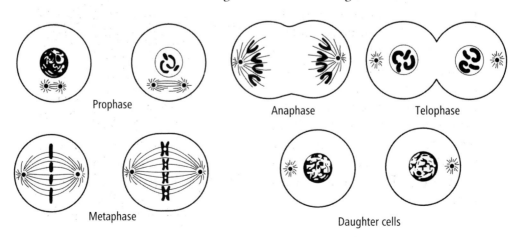

2 Tissues

A collection of cells with a common structure and function are called tissue. DNA will supply genetic material to determine the type of tissue formed. There are four main types of tissue in the human body – epithelial tissue, connective tissue, muscle tissue and nervous tissue.

Epithelial tissue

Epithelial tissue covers and protects the external and internal surfaces of the body. The cells form sheets of tissue and have various shapes depending on their function. Epithelial tissue is classified by the shape of the cell:

- Simple epithelium: a single layer of cells forming a smooth membrane suitable for diffusion, osmosis, filtration and secretion. In some cilia – small hairlike projections – are present to help move substances along, i.e. bronchus. The cells may be flat, cube or column shaped.

Simple epithelium (a) squamous, (b) cuboidal and (c) columnar ((i) ciliated and (ii) non-ciliated)

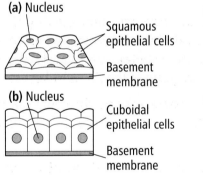
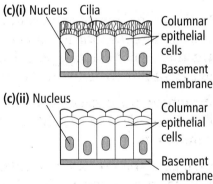

- Stratified epithelium: the stratified epithelium has at least two layers of cells of different shapes. The deep layers are column shape (columnar epithelium) that flatten (squamous epithelium) as they reach the surface. Stratified epithelium is able to withstand some wear and tear in order to protect underlying structures, for example skin tissue.

Stratified epithelium

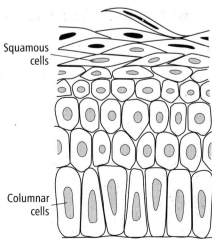

- Transitional epithelium: transitional epithelium is composed of several layers of tear-shaped cells. It is able to stretch without gaps appearing and this lining is found in the urinary bladder and ureters.

Transitional epithelium

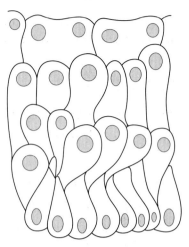

Modified epithelium

- Glandular epithelium: this layer of epithelium has glandular cells that lie within the lining. The glands may be endocrine (i.e. secreting hormones) or exocrine (i.e. secreting mucous, sweat, oil, milk, saliva and digestive enzymes).
- Pseudostratified columnar epithelium: columns of epithelium line the ducts of many glands. The nuclei of the cells are at different heights giving the impression of a multi-layered lining. In the upper respiratory tract this layer of epithelium will also contain goblet cells and cilia, which use a sweeping action to trap and remove foreign bodies.

Glandular epithelium

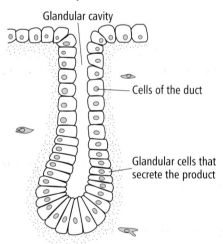

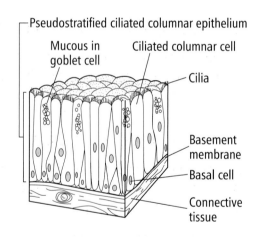

Connective tissue

Connective tissue is the most common type of tissue in the body as it is used to join, connect and support all the different structures. It is the major energy-storing and transport tissue in the body. The types of connective tissue are as follows.

Areolar connective tissue

This connective tissue is found in almost every part of the body. It contains cells called fibrocytes, yellow elastic fibres, white fibres, blood vessels and fat.

Adipose tissue

Adipose or fatty tissue contains fat globules and is found wherever there is areolar tissue. It is present under the skin and it provides insulation to reduce heat loss.

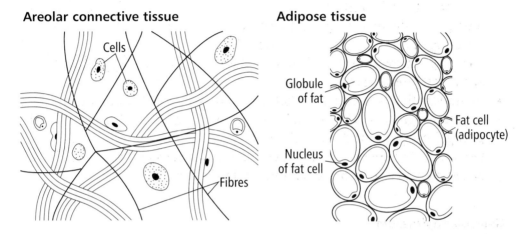

Areolar connective tissue

Cells

Fibres

Adipose tissue

Globule of fat

Fat cell (adipocyte)

Nucleus of fat cell

Dense regular connective tissue

Strong, dense connective cells form white fibrous tissue to create ligaments, periosteum and muscle fascia of the skeletal and muscle system. It also forms the outer protective layer of the brain and the kidneys.

Elastic connective tissue

This yellow connective tissue has elastic fibres that are capable of extension and recall. It is found in organs that require movement to function, particularly the arteries and lungs.

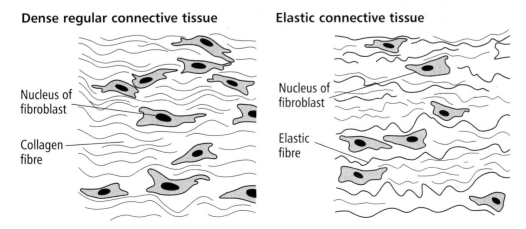

Dense regular connective tissue

Nucleus of fibroblast

Collagen fibre

Elastic connective tissue

Nucleus of fibroblast

Elastic fibre

Cartilage

Cartilage has a solid matrix (enclosed substance) and is therefore much stronger than other connective tissue. Cells of cartilage are called chondrocytes (kon-drō-sīts). Cartliage contains collagen and elastic fibres and has a covering of connective tissue called the perichondrium (per'-I-KON-drē-um). There are three different types of cartilage tissue:

- Hyaline cartilage: found in joints and the larynx, trachea and bronchi.

- White fibrocartilage: white connective tissue found between the vertebrae, knee and shoulder joints.

- Elastic cartilage: yellow elastic fibres run through the matrix, found in the epiglottis and ear lobe (pinna).

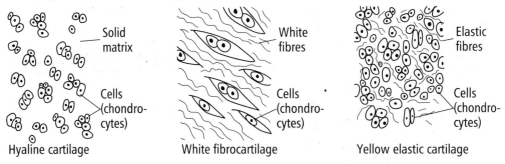

Hyaline cartilage — Solid matrix — Cells (chondrocytes)

White fibrocartilage — White fibres — Cells (chondrocytes)

Yellow elastic cartilage — Elastic fibres — Cells (chondrocytes)

Blood

Blood is a fluid connective tissue. The liquid matrix is called plasma and this contains water and dissolved nutrients, gases, hormones, salts, enzymes and waste. The plasma also transports red and white blood cells and platelets.

Lymph

Lymph is also a fluid connective tissue. It transports cells and chemicals from one part of the body to another.

Blood tissue

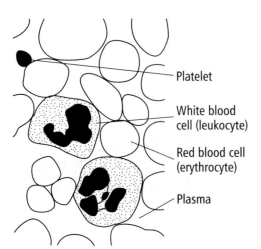

- Platelet
- White blood cell (leukocyte)
- Red blood cell (erythrocyte)
- Plasma

Lymphoid tissue (spleen) reticular cells have interlacing fibres that provide a network for support and strength

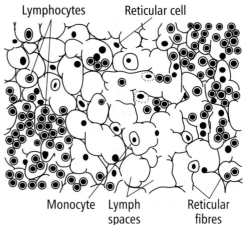

Lymphocytes   Reticular cell

Monocyte   Lymph spaces   Reticular fibres

Bone tissue

Bone is a very hard connective tissue. There are two types of bone tissue that make up the skeletal system:

- Compact: which to the naked eye looks solid but is made up of a well-defined structure called the Haversian system containing the lamellae, lacunae, canaliculi and a central canal.

- Spongy (or cancellous): this bone tissue has a honeycomb appearance and contains red bone marrow.

Haversian system – compact bone

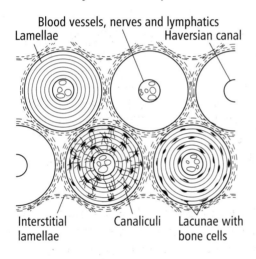

Lamellae
Blood vessels, nerves and lymphatics
Haversian canal

Interstitial lamellae
Canaliculi
Lacunae with bone cells

Spongy (cancellous) bone

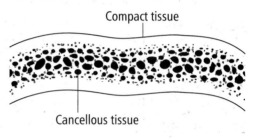

Compact tissue

Cancellous tissue

Muscle tissue

The cells of muscle tissue are adapted to generate force of varying degrees. Muscle tissue is divided into three groups, as follows.

Skeletal muscle

Also known as striated, striped or voluntary muscle (striated muscle is known as voluntary because it may be controlled by conscious thought). The fibres are long and cylindrical and usually attached to bone by a fibrous tissue called the tendon. They are used for motion, position and production of heat.

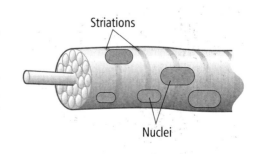

Striations

Nuclei

Smooth muscle

This is also known as involuntary or plain muscle. The fibres are spindle-shaped and are found in the walls of hollow organs. They provide motion through the hollow organs, i.e. the gastrointestinal tract. Smooth muscle cannot be controlled by conscious thought.

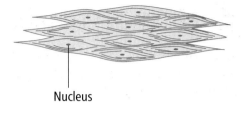

Nucleus

Cardiac muscle

Cardiac muscle is only found in the wall of the heart and the junction where major vessels enter or leave the heart. The muscle fibres are striated but unlike skeletal muscle have branches to interconnect. The branches connect at areas of thickened plasma membrane called intercalated discs. Cardiac muscle is involuntary muscle.

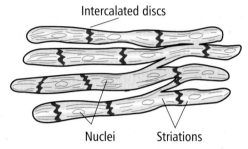

Intercalated discs

Nuclei   Striations

Nervous tissue

The nervous system is comprised of two types of nerve tissue – neurons and neurogia. The structure of neurons is detailed in Chapter 4.

Organs and systems

Organs are the collection of different tissues working together to carry out a specific function. Organs that work together to carry out functions create a system. In anatomy and physiology the body is divided into systems to allow a systematic approach to the study of the human body:

- Skeletal system
- Muscular system
- Nervous system
- Cardiovascular system
- Respiratory system
- Digestive system
- Genital-urinary system
- Lymphatic and immune system.

The individual systems carry out specific functions, but all systems need to function in harmony to maintain homeostasis.

3 Homeostasis

Homeostasis is the process of automatic and self-regulating mechanisms necessary to maintain the constant conditions needed for normal body function, despite any changes that may occur in the environment inside or outside of the body.

The internal environment of the body means the stable conditions that are necessary for all cells to survive and function. The trillions of body cells are surrounded by interstitial fluid containing nutrients and oxygen. The fluid flows around the body removing waste products from the cells and it also maintains the correct body temperature of 37 degrees centigrade. Chemical processes require enzymes to assist the body functions and they require set temperature and acidity levels in order to operate. All of the body's organs communicate and work together to help maintain the constancy of the internal environment.

The external environment relates to conditions outside the human body including the sociological and psychological factors that affect our everyday lives. Homeostasis enables humans to live in a variety of climates and conditions from hot deserts to Arctic ice fields. The body has mechanisms to help us flee from danger and survive trauma and stress. The study of homeostasis must therefore take into account all aspects of a person's biological, psychological and social environment.

Homeostasis changes to maintain the internal environment to within a narrow range of normal parameters. Homeostasis is therefore termed a dynamic process. The body makes constant adjustments to maintain 'dynamic equilibrium'. If homeostasis is not maintained it may result in illness, disease or death. Healthcare interventions may be required to help re-establish homeostasis.

Maintaining homeostasis

The organs within the body have one or more mechanisms to help regulate homeostatic control. The nervous system and the endocrine system control and regulate most of the mechanisms with the use of nerve impulses and hormones. The mechanisms needed for homeostasis are:

- Transport system: the respiratory, gastrointestinal, renal and cardiovascular systems communicate with the external environment supplying information and nutrients, water, oxygen and waste products to be transported to relevant organs.

- Detectors: the nervous system has receptors to detect any changes in the internal or external environment. Chemical changes are detected in cells to indicate low or high oxygen and carbon dioxide levels. Glands of the endocrine system detect changes in hormone levels, sending information called input to the relevant hormone control centre.

- Effectors: organs respond to messages from the detector. Nearly every organ in the body is an effector and is able to produce a response necessary to facilitate change.

- Regulators: the control systems include the nervous and endocrine systems. They make sure that the mechanisms of detectors and effectors work and that time of response is appropriate, with nerve impulses creating rapid responses compared with the slower response to hormones.

Regulating homeostasis

When an imbalance occurs in any cell the automatic and self-regulating mechanism will come into effect to counteract and rebalance. This process is called negative feedback.

Negative feedback

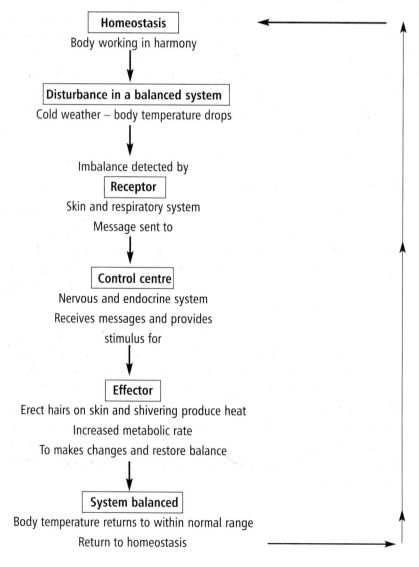

| Homeostasis |
| Body working in harmony |

| Disturbance in a balanced system |
Cold weather – body temperature drops

Imbalance detected by
| Receptor |
Skin and respiratory system
Message sent to

| Control centre |
Nervous and endocrine system
Receives messages and provides
stimulus for

| Effector |
Erect hairs on skin and shivering produce heat
Increased metabolic rate
To makes changes and restore balance

| System balanced |
Body temperature returns to within normal range
Return to homeostasis

Positive feedback systems

Positive feedback works in a similar way to negative feedback except that the changes made have the effect of inducing further change to occur. This system has a positive effect in situations such as childbirth where it maintains contractions of the uterus, but most positive feedback causes harm if homeostatic balances remain disrupted, for example shock due to severe bleeding. Positive feedback acts to continue an imbalance rather than stopping/reversing it.

Homeostasis and health

When the body is in homeostasis the trillions of cells within the body function effectively and provide a healthy internal environment. If this healthy balance is disturbed it may have serious consequences for the cells, resulting in disorders, disease or death.

Healthcare professionals need to know how the body functions and the range of normal values necessary to maintain homeostasis if they are to detect and intervene to restore imbalances. Client care must be based on a holistic approach to disease or disorders with an understanding of how all organs may be affected if an imbalance occurs. Assessing, planning and implementing care needs to be based on the biological, psychological and social needs of a client to ensure a return to optimum health or the maintaining of quality of life for clients with terminal illness.

The terms used to describe an imbalance of homeostasis are:

- Disorder: an abnormality of the function of organs or systems.

- Disease: an illness that affects one part of the body (localised), or several parts, or the whole body (systemic). Some diseases alter the functions or structure of the body in specific ways, producing changes called signs and symptoms. Signs are changes in the body that may be seen or measured, such as a rash or high temperature. Symptoms are changes that the client notices, for example pain or tiredness.

Diseases and disorders may be inherited or acquired. The body has its own defence system (the immune system) to fight against disease and disorders, but many diseases occur following abuse caused by a person's own behaviour and environment. The body requires a balanced diet, clean air, exercise and rest to maintain quality of life and optimum health. Behaviours that abuse the homeostatic processes, such as smoking, alcohol/drug abuse, lack of exercise, poor diet and stressful or polluted environments will result in disease if the abuse continues over a period of time. Therefore, lifestyles are an important factor in homeostasis.

Further reading

Clancy, J., McVicar, A. and Baird, N. (2001) *Fundamentals of Physiological Homeostasis for Perioperative Practitioners*. Routledge, London.

Clarke, L., Sachs B. and Ford-Sumner, S. (2000) *Health and Social Care for Advanced GNVQ*, 3rd edn. Nelson Thornes, Cheltenham.

Taylor, C., Lillis, C. and LeMone, P. (1997) *Fundamentals of Nursing: The Art and Science of Nursing Care*, 3rd edn. Nelson Thornes, Cheltenham.

Vellacott, J. and Side, S. (1998) *Understanding Advanced Human Biology*. Hodder and Stoughton, London.

Chapter 2
The skeletal system and movement

National unit specification
These are the topics you will be studying for this unit.

1 The skeletal system and types of bones

2 Bone cells and bone growth

3 The axial skeleton

4 The appendicular skeleton

5 Diseases and disorders of the skeletal system

6 Joints

7 Types of movement

8 Diseases and disorders of joints

9 The muscular system

10 The sliding-filament mechanism of muscle contraction

11 Metabolism of skeletal muscle

12 Diseases and disorders of muscles

Diagrams to practise:
Skeleton – naming the main bones
Types of bones
Structure of the long bone
Compact bone
Trabecular bone
Spinal column
Vertebrae
Types of joints
Knee joint
Organisation of skeletal muscle
Sliding-filament mechanism

Your assessment may include time-constraint tests, the presentation of experiments in the form of written reports, and case studies of specific diseases or disorders affecting the skeletal system.

Homeostasis

The skeletal system is made up of bones that support and protect internal organs of the body. Bones store calcium which is necessary for many body functions.

Skin:
Bones provide support and joints allow movement.

Muscle system:
Bones provide the base for muscle attachment. Muscle obtains calcium for movement.

Nervous system:
Provides protection for the brain and spinal column. Needs calcium to function.

Endocrine system:
Calcium is needed for the function of many hormones.

Cardiovascular system:
Red blood cells are formed in bone. Heart muscle requires calcium.

Lymphatic system:
White blood cells are made in bone marrow.

Respiratory system:
Rib cage protects the lungs.

Digestive system:
Teeth prepare food before swallowing. Rib cage protects the upper Gastrointestinal tract and liver.

Urinary system:
Ribs help protect the kidneys. Pelvis protects the bladder

Reproductive system:
Pelvis protects the ovaries, fallopian tubes and uterus.
Calcium is needed during lactation.

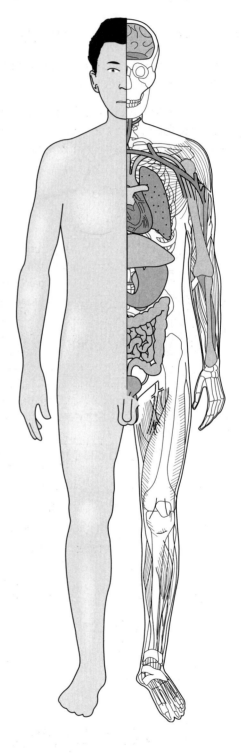

1 The skeletal system and types of bones

Anatomy of the skeleton

To demonstrate an understanding of the anatomy of the skeleton you will be required to learn the names of the main bones in the human body.

It is difficult to understand the relationship of the bones when viewed in diagrammatic form. Use the anatomical models available at college to help you gain a deeper understanding of the structure of the skeleton.

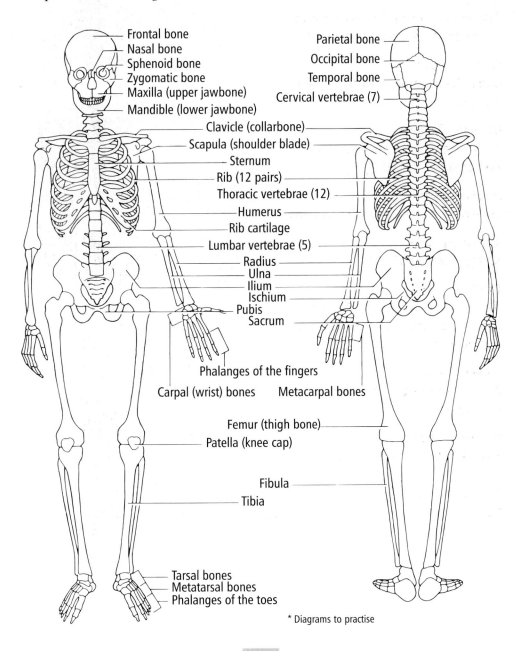

Frontal bone
Nasal bone
Sphenoid bone
Zygomatic bone
Maxilla (upper jawbone)
Mandible (lower jawbone)

Parietal bone
Occipital bone
Temporal bone
Cervical vertebrae (7)

Clavicle (collarbone)
Scapula (shoulder blade)
Sternum
Rib (12 pairs)
Thoracic vertebrae (12)
Humerus
Rib cartilage
Lumbar vertebrae (5)
Radius
Ulna
Ilium
Ischium
Pubis
Sacrum

Phalanges of the fingers
Carpal (wrist) bones   Metacarpal bones

Femur (thigh bone)
Patella (knee cap)

Fibula
Tibia

Tarsal bones
Metatarsal bones
Phalanges of the toes

* Diagrams to practise

The skeletal system

The skeletal system consists of:

- All of the bones in the body (the bony skeleton).

- All associated cartilages and joints.

Functions of the skeletal system

- Support: it supports the soft body tissue thus allowing us to stand.

- Assisting with body movement: it provides attachment areas for skeletal muscle and joints for flexibility.

- Protection: the skeleton helps to protect soft vital organs, e.g. the skull (cranial bones) protects the brain, the rib cage protects the heart and lungs.

- Storing minerals and fats: the skeleton also stores large amounts of calcium and phosphorus.

- Storing cells needed to manufacture blood cells: the red bone marrow found in certain bones produces red and white blood cells and platelets.

Types of bones

The bony skeleton consists of approximately 206 bones. Bones are classified by their shape and location. There are five main types of bone:

- Long bones: found in the limbs, these are cylindrical in shape.

- Short bones: square or rectangular in shape and found in the wrist or foot.

- Flat bones: these are thin and provide a surface area for muscle attachment.

Long bone: right femur (anterior view)

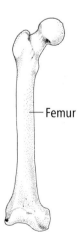

Femur

Short bones in the left wrist (anterior view)

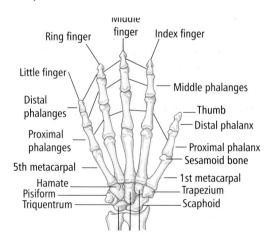

Flat bones: ribs

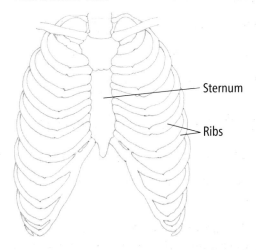

Sternum

Ribs

Irregular bones of the spinal column

- Irregular bones: these have complex shapes and are found in the face and spine.

Cervical vertebrae

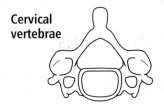

Sesamoid bone: patella

- Sesamoid bones: these are found in tendons that have excessive friction, such as the soles of the feet (where the number of sesamoid bones varies) or the kneecap (patella).

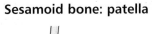
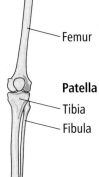

Femur

Patella

Tibia

Fibula

The bones of the skeleton are divided into two main groups:

- The axial skeleton: which contains bones of the axis or upper parts of the body.

Pelvic (hip) girdle
  Hip, pelvic, or coxal bone
Lower limbs
  Femur
  Fibula
  Tibia
  Patella
  Tarsals
  Metatarsals
  Phalanges

Pectoral (shoulder) girdles
  Clavicle
  Scapula
Upper limbs
  Humerus
  Ulna
  Radius
  Carpals
  Metacarpals
  Phalanges

- The appendicular skeleton: which contains 126 bones of the shoulder, pelvis and limbs.

Skull
  Cranium
  Face
Hyoid
Auditory ossicles
Vertebral column
Thorax
  Sternum
  Ribs

Structure of bone

Bone is made of connective tissue and its strength comes from the calcium phosphate and calcium carbonate in the matrix. The main strength of bone is in the dense outer layer which is made of mineralised tissue called compact bone. Although bones are strong they are relatively light because of the presence of the spongy internal bone tissue called cancellous or trabecular bone.

Section through a long bone

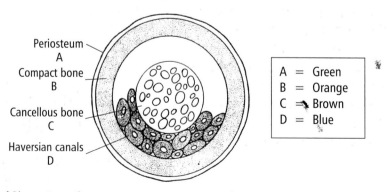

Periosteum
A
Compact bone
B
Cancellous bone
C
Haversian canals
D

A = Green
B = Orange
C = Brown
D = Blue

* Diagram to practise

Compact bone

Compact bone is the hard, dense outer shell of a bone. Although the outer shell may look smooth, it has a complex structure that consists of minute cylindrical structures called osteons or Haversian systems.

The Haversian system has a central canal that runs along the axis of the bone. The canal is used to convey blood vessels, lymph vessels and neurons into the bone tissue. Side canals radiate out to allow blood flow through the compact bone structure. There are also very small channels called canaliculi that are filled with tissue fluid. The canaliculi expand to contain bone cells (called osteocytes). Osteocytes receive nutrients from the tissue fluid.

Blood vessels in bone come from the periosteum – the outer covering of bone. Compact bone is perforated by nutrient foramina (windows) that allow vessels to enter and drain tissue fluid. Branches of these blood vessels also supply the underlying spongy (trabecular) bone and bone marrow.

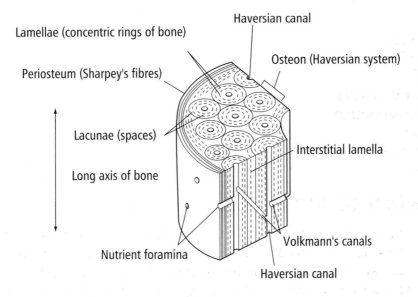

Lamellae (concentric rings of bone)
Haversian canal
Periosteum (Sharpey's fibres)
Osteon (Haversian system)
Lacunae (spaces)
Interstitial lamella
Long axis of bone
Nutrient foramina
Volkmann's canals
Haversian canal

Trabecular bone

Trabecular bone looks like a sponge and consists of a network of minute archways and beams that provide strength to the bone but also help to reduce bone weight. The hollows in trabecular bone before birth and in infancy contain red bone marrow. In adults they are filled with yellow bone marrow which is a fatty substance.

Trabecular structure of a spongy bone

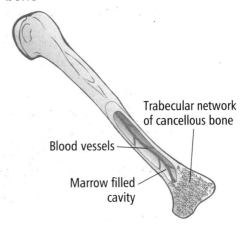

Trabecular network of cancellous bone
Blood vessels
Marrow filled cavity

* Diagram to practise

2 Bone cells and bone growth

Bone cells are classified according to their function. The types of bone cells are:

- Osteogenic cells (os′-tē-ō-JEN-ik): these are stem cells, basic cells from which specialised cells are formed. They are found in the periosteum and endosteum. They are able to develop into osteoblasts or osteoclasts necessary following injury or mechanical stress.

- Osteoblasts (OS-tē-ō-blasts): these are young osteocytes and they produce new bone. They are responsible for producing calcium deposits and also new bone following bone injury.

- Osteocytes (OS-tē-ō-sits′): these are the main cells of developed bone and they maintain the protein and mineral matrix. These cells have an elongated body with thin tendrils.

- Osteoclasts (OSt-ē-ō-clasts′): these are phagocytic cells responsible for removing minerals from the protein matrix and rebuilding bone where necessary. These cells are able to create microscopic tunnels within the bone.

Types of bone cell

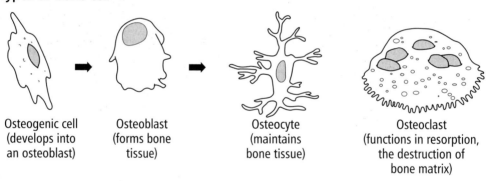

Osteogenic cell
(develops into
an osteoblast)

Osteoblast
(forms bone
tissue)

Osteocyte
(maintains
bone tissue)

Osteoclast
(functions in resorption,
the destruction of
bone matrix)

Bone growth

The formation and growth of bones begins in the fetus and continues until late teens or early twenties.

In the fetus the process of bone development is called primary ossification. The first stage of development involves the formation of cartilage or fibrous membranes that act as a framework for the developing bone. As the fetus develops, the cartilage-forming cells are destroyed and osteoblasts and osteoclasts form. At birth the long bones are still largely made of cartilage and the baby will not be able to weight bear until further ossification takes place.

Bone growth at the epiphysial plate

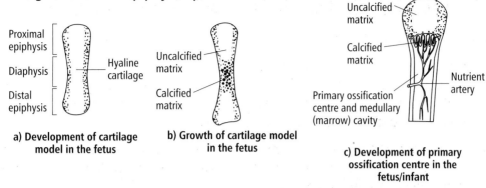

a) Development of cartilage model in the fetus

b) Growth of cartilage model in the fetus

c) Development of primary ossification centre in the fetus/infant

Secondary ossification occurs during early childhood. The area between the epiphysis and the bony shaft is called the epiphyseal plate and this produces further bone formation. The epiphyseal plate will continue to produce new bone until the end of the growth period. It will then disappear and growth of the bone will cease.

Bone will continue to alter throughout a person's lifetime as old bone is renewed and injured bone is replaced.

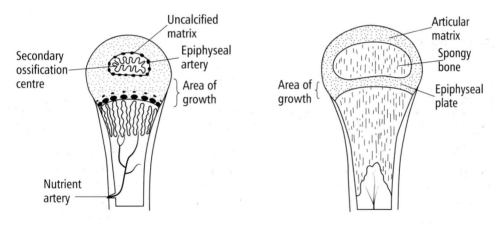

d) Development of secondary ossification centre in epiphysis during childhood

e) Formation of articular cartilage and epiphyseal plate during childhood

Hormones and bone growth

Growth hormone, controlled by the hypothalamus and produced in the anterior pituitary gland, is the main hormone involved with the stimulation of bone growth at the epiphyseal plate.

Other hormones that also stimulate bone growth are thyroid hormones and the sex hormones oestrogen and testosterone.

A deficiency (hyposecretion) or overproduction (hypersecretion) of growth hormone before bone growth is complete will influence the height of a person. Hyposecretion will limit growth (dwarfism) and hypersecretion will cause gigantism.

3 Axial skeleton

The axial skeleton consists of bones that form the vertical axis of the body.

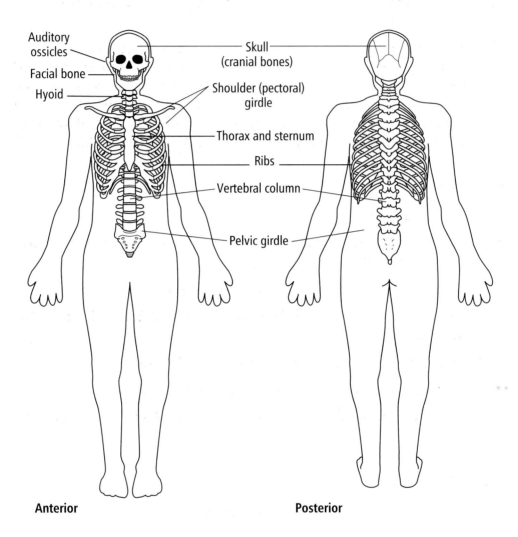

Auditory ossicles

Facial bone

Hyoid

Skull (cranial bones)

Shoulder (pectoral) girdle

Thorax and sternum

Ribs

Vertebral column

Pelvic girdle

Anterior

Posterior

The skull

The skull consists of flat or irregular bones. There are eight cranial bones that protect the brain and 14 facial bones. The bones of the skull develop separately but fuse together as they mature. The only movable joint in a fully formed skull is the mandible (lower jaw).

The cranial bones (collectively called the cranium) enclose and protect the brain. In a baby the cranial bones are divided by membrane-filled spaces called fontanels (fon-ta-NELZ). These spaces will eventually be replaced by bone and will fuse together, connected by serrated joints or sutures. A suture (SOO-chur) is an immovable joint made of connective tissue and it does not allow movement of the bone. Serrated joints/sutures are only present in the skull.

Functions of the skull

- Cranial bones protect the brain.
- Bony eye sockets help to protect the eye against injury and provide an area for the attachment of the eye muscles.
- The temporal bone protects the inner structures of the ear.
- Some facial bones contain cavities called sinuses which assist in producing vocal sounds.
- Posterior nasal bones help to maintain the nasal airway.
- The mandible and maxilla provide anchorage for the teeth.
- The mandible is the only movable bone of the skull and allows food to be chewed.

Views of the skull

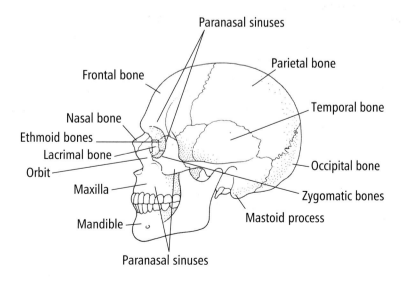

Cranial bones

Frontal bone

- This bone forms the forehead, roof of the eye sockets and the front part of the base of the skull.

- Vessels and nerves pass through a notch in the front area of the eye socket.

- Above the eyebrows the frontal bone is hollow and forms two air-filled spaces called the frontal sinuses.

Parietal bones (pa-RĪ-e-tal)

- There are two parietal bones.

- They meet at the top of the skull at a suture called the sagittal suture (SAJ-I-tal).

- They form most of the roof and sides of the cranial cavity.

Temporal bones

- There are two temporal bones.

- They are found at the sides of the skull and they form part of the cranial floor and contain the ear canal.

- The temporal bone is divided into four parts:
  - Squamous part: joins the parietal bone and also the zygomatic process (facial bones).
  - Tympanic part: contains the external ear canal.
  - Mastoid process: a small projection behind the ear that contains tiny air cells.
  - Petrous portion: contains semicircular canals of the inner ear.

Occipital bone (ok-SIP-I-tal)

- This forms the back of the skull and the major portion of the base.

- The foramen magnum passes through the occipital bone. Within this foramen is the medulla oblongata that connects to the spinal cord and spinal arteries.

- On either side of the foramen magnum are oval processes called occipital condyles which join with the first part of the spine.

Facial bones

Mandible

- This is the lower jaw and it forms the chin.

- It contains the lower teeth.

- The angle of the jaw is created where the body of the mandible curves up to the ramus.

- The ramus provides attachment muscle and also articulates with the temporal bone.

- The temporo-mandibular joint is a complex synovial joint that allows you to open and close your mouth and to move your jaw sideways, backwards and forwards.

Maxilla

- The maxilla develops from two halves called maxillae (mak-SIL-ē). They will normally fuse in the midline before birth.

- An alveolar ridge contains the upper teeth.

- This bone forms part of the orbit of the eye and the hard palate of the mouth.

- Underneath the orbits (eye sockets) there is a large air space within the bone known as the maxillary sinus.

Lacrimal bones (LAK-ri-mal)

- The two small lacrimal bones form part of the outer (medial) wall of the orbit.

- The drainage ducts for tears pass through the lacrimal bones to the nasal cavity.

Zygomatic bones

- These are also called cheekbones.

- They form the floor and lateral wall of each orbit.

Nasal bones

- The bridge of the nose is formed by the two nasal bones.

- The floor of the nose is formed by a triangular-shaped bone called the vomer (VŌ-mer). This bone forms part of the wall that divides the nose.

- Two scroll-like bones, the inferior nasal conchae, project into the nasal cavity and assist in the filtration of air as it passes through to the lungs.

- Most of the nose is made from cartilage not bone.

Paranasal sinuses

- The sinuses are lined with a mucous membrane that is continuous with the lining of the nasal cavity.

- The sinuses produce mucous that drains into the nasal cavity.

- The condition known as sinusitis is caused by inflammation of the membranes as a result of an allergic reaction or infection.

Orbit

- The orbit is the eye socket.

- It is cone shaped and designed to protect the eye.

Ethmoid bones

- These are two small bones found in the centre of the orbits.

- The bones contain air spaces that form the ethmoidal sinuses.

Vertebral column

Vertebral (spinal) column

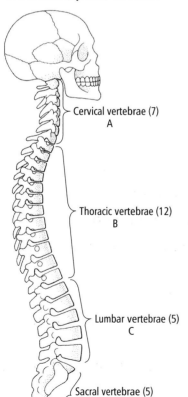

Cervical vertebrae (7)
A

Thoracic vertebrae (12)
B

Lumbar vertebrae (5)
C

Sacral vertebrae (5)
D

Coccygeal vertebrae (4)
E

A	=	Green
B	=	Orange
C	=	Brown
D	=	Blue
E	=	Pink

* Diagram to practise

The vertebral column (spine) is responsible for:

- Supporting the body.

- Providing attachment for muscle.

- Protecting the spinal cord.

- Acting as a shock absorber.

There are 33 vertebrae (VER-te-brē) in the vertebral column, interlinked with cartilage, making it a flexible structure. The general structure of each vertebra is similar, with slight differences according to their position and function in the vertebral column.

Curvature of the spinal column

- In a baby the spine has a C-shaped curve.

- As the child develops the spine becomes a distinctive S-shape.

- The curves of the spine help to ensure that the centre of gravity remains over the pelvis when a person is standing up.

- If the centre of gravity is distorted it will lead to lateral curves and incorrect posture which may require physiotherapy or surgery to correct.

Curves of the spine

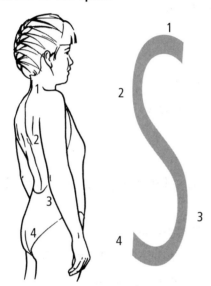 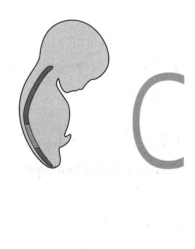

Vertebrae

- The vertebrae are numbered from the top to the bottom.

- Each vertebra has a body called a centrum and a neural arch.

- The body and arch enclose a round opening, called the neural canal or vertebrae foramen, which carries the spinal canal.

- Arising from the arch are processes or projections.

- The spinous process projects out from the back of the arch and is used for tendon attachment.

- The transverse processes project out from the sides of the arch and are also used for tendon attachment.

- The superior and inferior articular processes, pointing upwards and downwards, form joints with other vertebrae.

The five different vertebrae (transverse view/side view)

Atlas and axis

Cervical vertebrae

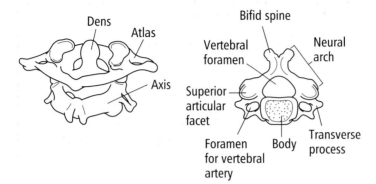

Thoracic vertebrae

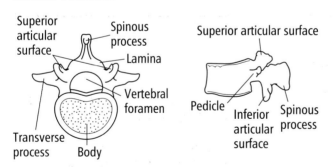

Lumbar vertebrae

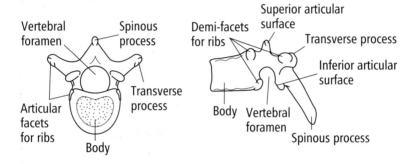

Sacral vertebrae

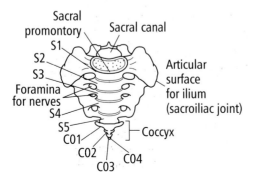

The vertebra are divided into five areas.

Vertebrae

Vertebrae	Number of vertebrae	Functions
Cervical: in the neck region	7	First two vertebrae are called the atlas and axis – they allow nodding of the head
Thoracic: chest	12	Larger and stronger than cervical vertebrae. They join (articulate) with the ribs
Lumbar: loin	5	Largest and strongest vertebrae. They support the upper body and are adapted for the attachment of large back muscles
Sacral	5	The five sacral vertebrae are fused together to form a triangular bone called the sacrum (SÀ-krum). It supports the pelvic girdle
Coccyx (KOK-siks)	4	The four bones are fused to form the coccygeal (kok-SIJ-ē-al) vertebrae: The bones are relatively small and have no special function

Intervertebral joints

To allow movement of the spine there are synovial joints and intervertebral discs between the vertebrae.

- Synovial joints lie between the superior articular process of one vertebra and the inferior articular process of the vertebra directly above.

- Between every two vertebrae connected by a synovial joint there is an opening called the intervertebral foramen that allows nerves to emerge from the spinal cord.

Anterior view of intervertebral joints, discs and ligaments

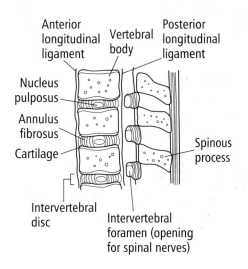

Anterior longitudinal ligament
Vertebral body
Posterior longitudinal ligament
Nucleus pulposus
Annulus fibrosus
Cartilage
Spinous process
Intervertebral disc
Intervertebral foramen (opening for spinal nerves)

Intervertebral discs

- There is a cartilaginous joint between the vertebra to help the spine to act as a shock absorber and to permit movement.
- The joint is made from a disc of fibrocartilage that has a soft gelatinous interior. The fibrous outer cover is called the annulus fibrosis and the highly elastic soft centre is called the nucleus pulposus.
- The intervertebral disc becomes compressed and absorbs the pressure from body weight. The outer annulus fibrosis ensures that the soft centre stays in the correct place and does not leak.
- If the nucleus pulposus does escape from the outer covering it is termed 'a slipped disc'.

Thorax

The thorax refers to all anatomy of the chest. The thoracic cage is the bony cage made up of the following.

- The sternum or breastbone: consisting of three parts:
  - The upper part is called the manubrium (ma-NOO-brĕ-um).
  - The centre is called the body.
  - The lowest, smallest part is called the xiphoid process (ZĬ-foyd) or xiphisternum.
- Ribs: 12 pairs of flat bones connected to the synovial joints of the spine. The first set of 10 ribs are also connected to the sternum at the front of the thoracic cage. They are connected by costal cartilage.
- Costal cartilage: this joins the ribs at the front, and the lower edge of the rib cage. This is called the costal margin.
- Thoracic vertebrae: forms part of the spine that is the thoracic curve and consists of 12 vertebrae.

The thoracic cage protects the organs in the thoracic cavity and upper abdominal cavity. It also provides support for the bones of the shoulder and upper limbs.

Rib and thorax

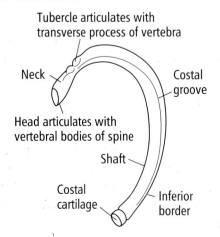

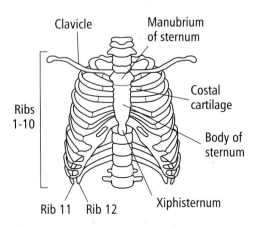

4 The appendicular skeleton

Anterior view of appendicular skeleton

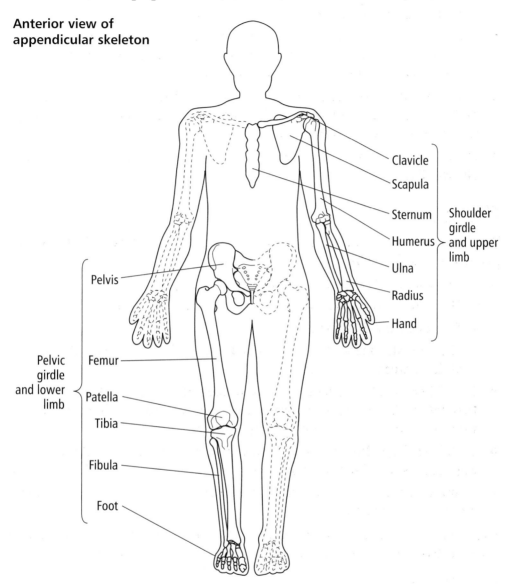

Pectoral girdle

The pectoral girdle (PEK-tō-ral) is also known as the shoulder girdle and relates to the bones that attach the upper limbs (arms) to the axial skeleton. There are two bones in the pectoral girdle:

- Clavicle (KLAV-I-kul) or collarbone: this is connected to the sternum and to the scapula.

- Scapula (SCAP-yoo-la) or shoulder blade: this is a large, flat, triangular bone situated in the upper part of the back. It is connected to the clavicle and has a cup-shaped cavity (the glenoid fossa) that holds the head of the humerus (upper arm bone) to form the shoulder joint. The scapula is a flat bone designed for muscle attachment.

Upper limbs

The upper limb (arm) consists of 30 different bones:

- Humerus (HYOO-mer-us).

- Ulna and radius.

- Carpals: eight wrist bones.

- Metacarpals: five bones of the palm of the hand.

- Phalanges (fa-LAN-jēz): 14 finger bones.

Clavicle and scapula

(diagram: Scapula, Clavicle, Humerus)

Humerus

- The longest and largest bone of the upper limbs.

- The proximal end (shoulder) is rounded, covered with cartilage and called the head of the humerus.

- At the elbow the trochlea (TRŌK-lē-a), a spoon-shaped surface, articulates with the ulna. The capitulum (ka-PIT-yoo-lum) is a small round knob that articulates with the head of the radius.

- The body of the humerus has a v-shaped area, the deltoid tuberosity, used for attachment of the deltoid muscle.

Ulna and radius

Ulna

- This is on the little-finger side of the forearm (medial aspect).

- It is longer than the radius.

- At the top (proximal) end is the olecranon that forms the prominence of the elbow and acts to prevent the hyperextension (over-extension) of the elbow.

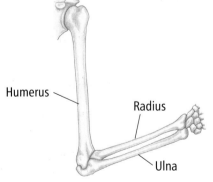

Ulna and radius

(diagram labels: Humerus, Radius, Ulna)

- The joint between the ulna and the humerus is a hinge joint allowing movement in one direction or plane.

- The shaft of the ulna provides attachment for muscles of the forearm.

- A stynoid process is at the distal (lower) end of the ulna and provides attachment for the wrist muscle.

Radius

- This is found on the thumb side of the forearm (lateral aspect).

- The proximal (top) end is rounded and covered with articular cartilage and is called the head of the radius.

- The head of the radius articulates with the humerus.

- Below the head the radial tuberosity provides attachment for the bicep muscles.

- The shaft provides attachment for muscle and is narrow and rounded in shape. The radius widens at the lower end and there is a lateral concave surface that articulates with carpal bones.

Carpals

- The eight bones in the wrist are called carpal bones.

- The carpals are held together by ligaments.

- The carpals are short bones arranged in two rows of four bones. Each bone is named according to its shape (see the diagram of the wrist below).

Metacarpals

- There are five metacarpal bones in the hand (the palm).

- The metacarpals are numbered 1 to 5 starting with the thumb or pollex.

- The heads of the metacarpals are visible when the hand is clenched and are commonly referred to as the knuckles.

- Each metacarpal consists of a proximal base and a distal head.

Bones of the wrist and hand

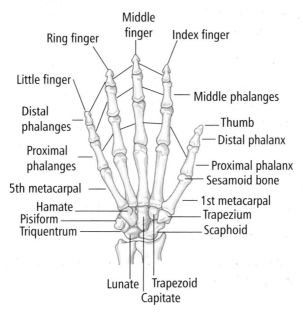

The phalanges

- The bones of the fingers are called the phalanges (fa-LAN-jēz).

- In the thumb there are two phalanges and in each finger there are three phalanges called the proximal, middle and distal phalanx (FĀ-lanks (singular)).

Pelvic girdle

The pelvic (hip) girdle joins the leg to the axial skeleton. The pelvic girdle is the site of the body's centre of gravity and provides strong support for the vertebral column. The bones which make up the pelvic girdle are the innominate or hip bones.

- Each hip bone consists of three separate bones: the ilium, the ischium and the pubis. These bones are fused together to form one large, robust, irregular bone.

- The hip bones are connected at the front at a joint called the pubic symphysis (PYOO-bik SIM-fi-sis).

- At the back (posterior) they unite with the sacrum at the sacroiliac joint.

- The bones form a basin-like structure called the pelvis.

- On the outer surface is a deep depression called the acetabulum that forms part of the hip joint.

- The ilium is the largest subdivision of the pelvic girdle. The upper border is called the iliac crest. The lower border has a notch called the greater sciatic notch (sī-AT-ik) through which the longest nerve, the sciatic nerve, passes.

- The ischium (IS-kē-um) is the lower (inferior) part of the hip.

- The pubis (PYOO-bis): the two pubic bones unite in the midline at the symphysis pubis to form the pubic arch.

Pelvic girdle: (a) female and (b) male

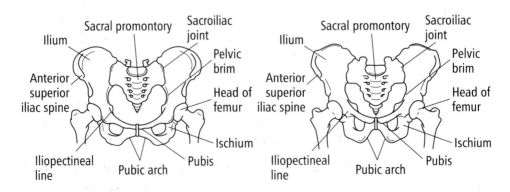

Differences between the female and male pelvis

The female pelvis has distinct differences to allow for childbirth.

Differences between male and female pelvis

	Female	Male
Bones	Lighter	Longer
Pelvic cavity	Shallow and round	Deep and more funnel-shaped
Sacrum	Broad and short, more concave at the front to make the pelvic area larger	Less concave, and the pelvis is narrower at the outlet
Pelvic brim	Oval	Heart-shaped
Pubic arch	The angle of the pubic bones make the pubic arch wider and the acetabula further apart (wider hips)	The angle of the pubic bones make the pubic arch narrower and their acetabula closer together

Lower limbs

Each of the two lower limbs (legs) are composed of 30 bones:

- Femur: the thigh bone.

- Patella: the knee cap.

- Tibia and fibula: the long bones between the knee and the ankle.

- Tarsals: the seven ankle bones.

- Metatarsals: five bones forming the central part of the foot.

- Phalanges: 14 bones in the toes.

Femur

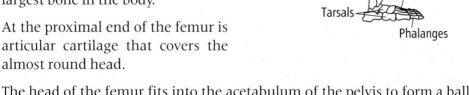

- This is the longest, strongest and largest bone in the body.

- At the proximal end of the femur is articular cartilage that covers the almost round head.

- The head of the femur fits into the acetabulum of the pelvis to form a ball and socket joint which enables movement in all planes.

- Below the head, at an angle of 135°, is the neck of the femur (an anatomical weak point, commonly fractured in the elderly (fractured hip)).

- The greater and lesser trochanter (troŏ-KAN-ter) are two large projections situated at the junction of the neck and the shaft of the femur. The trochanter give attachment to muscles of the thighs and buttocks.

- At the distal end of the femur are two projections called the medial condyle and lateral condyle. The ends of the condyle form the upper part of the knee joint.

Patella

The patella (knee cap) is a sesamoid bone, triangular in shape. Its functions are to:

- Protect the knee joint.

- Assist in the function of the thigh muscles (quadriceps femoris muscle).

- Maintain the position of tendons when the knee is bent (flexed).

Tibia and fibula

The tibia and fibula are the two long bones of the lower leg.

Tibia

- The tibia (shin bone) is the larger bone and is positioned medial to the fibula.

- The tibia articulates at the proximal end with the femur and fibula.

- The medial and lateral condyles are two prominences from the proximal end of the tibia that articulate with the condyles of the femur to form the knee joint.

- Below the tibial condyles is a prominence called the tibial tuberosity which is a point of attachment for the patella ligament.

- The shaft of the tibia is triangular in shape and the medial surface is a prominent crest that can be felt just under the skin.

- At the distal end of the tibia there is an articulating surface for the talus of the ankle that forms a prominence, the medial malleolus (ma-LĒ-ō-lus), which feels like a lump on the inside of the ankle.

Fibula

- The fibula is the lateral non-weight bearing bone. It is smaller than the tibia.

- The fibula articulates at the proximal end with the lateral condyle of the tibia.

- The shaft of the fibula provides muscle attachment.

- The fibular notch is found at the distal end and connects the tibia to the fibula.

- Also at the distal end of the fibula there is a projection called the lateral malleolus that articulates with the talus of the ankle (which feels like a lump on the outside of the ankle).

Tarsals

- The structure of the foot is similar to the hand.

- The seven short tarsals form the ankle and heel of the foot and support the body weight. The two posterior tarsals are called the talus and the calcaneus.

- The talus articulates with the tibia and fibula.

- The calcaneus (Kal-KĀ-nē-us) or heel bone provides attachment for the Achilles tendon and is the largest and strongest of the tarsals.

Metatarsals

- The five metatarsals are small long bones that form the instep or dorsum of the foot.

- The bones are numbered 1 to 5, the big toe being the first metatarsal.

- The proximal end articulates with the tarsals and the distal end with the phalanges.

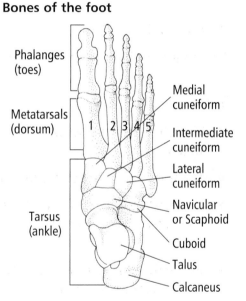

Bones of the foot

Phalanges (toes)

Metatarsals (dorsum)

Tarsus (ankle)

1 2 3 4 5

Medial cuneiform

Intermediate cuneiform

Lateral cuneiform

Navicular or Scaphoid

Cuboid

Talus

Calcaneus

Phalanges

- The 14 phalanges in the toes are arranged in the same way as the hand.

- The big or great toe has two phalanges; these are large and heavy to help support weight. The other four toes have three phalanges.

Arches of the foot

The foot has to be strong and flexible as it is designed to bear weight and provide leverage when walking. The bones of the foot are connected by ligaments and tendons, which create arches.

- The structure of an arch provides strength, flexibility and helps to absorb shocks.

- The arches are not rigid and are able to adapt their shape according to the surface being walked on.

- The foot has three arches: the medial arch, lateral arch and transverse arch.

- If the ligaments and tendons of the medial arch are damaged it may cause the height of the arch to fall and create the condition known as flatfoot.

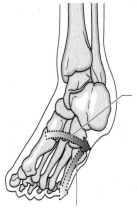

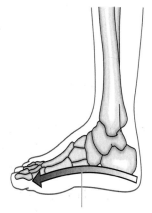

Transverse arch – between the medical and lateral aspects of the foot

Lateral longitudinal arch – on the little toe side of the foot

Medial longitudinal arch – the highest arch on the big toe side of the foot

5 Diseases and disorders of the skeletal system

Bunion (BUN-yun)

This is a deformity of the big toe often caused by a person wearing shoes that are tight around the toes. At the joints of the phalanges the fluid-filled sacs (bursae) become swollen (inflamed) and calluses may form.

Fractures

A cracked or broken bone is called a fracture. The continuity of the bone is disrupted as a result of excessive force.

There are different types of fractures depending upon the kind of force that has caused the trauma. Fractures are named according to specific features:

- Closed fracture: the bone is fractured but the overlying skin is intact.

- Open fracture: the broken ends of the fractured bone perforate the overlying skin.

- Compound fracture: more than one bone may be fractured, for example the tibia and fibula, and there will be more than one fracture – the bone being broken in several places (comminuted fracture).

- Partial or stress fracture: an incomplete break or crack across the bone. In children the fracture is called a greenstick fracture, similar to the damage caused if a young tree branch is bent.

Types of fractures

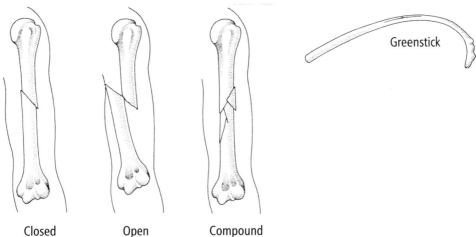

Closed   Open   Compound   Greenstick

- Pathological fracture: a fracture that is caused when bone disease is present, such as bone cancer. Fractures may occur with minimal force.

The healing process for bones will depend on the type of fracture, the treatment received and the general health of a person. The process of repair involves cells derived from the periosteum.

Herniated disc

If the fibrous ring of the intervertebral discs becomes weakened it may rupture allowing the inner gel to escape and herniate (protrude) from the disc. This may cause pressure or irritation on nearby spinal nerves, leading to mild to severe pain radiating down the leg on the side of the rupture. This condition is commonly known as a slipped disc and occurs most often in the lumbar region of the spinal column.

Kyphosis (kī-FŌ-sis)

This name is given to an extended curve of the thoracic vertebrae caused by degeneration of the invertebrae discs, rickets or poor posture. It is a relatively common condition in the elderly.

Lordosis (lor-DŌ-sis)

This condition is an exaggeration of the lumbar curve. Lordosis may be due to extreme obesity causing increased weight of the abdomen, or poor posture, rickets or tuberculosis of the spine.

Osteomyelitis (OŚ-tē-ōm-a-my-a-lī-tīs)

This condition occurs when bacteria invade the bone tissue. Bacteria may be spread to bone tissue by the bloodstream, during operations on bone, from neighbouring infected soft tissue or when a broken bone has penetrated through the skin (open fracture). The infected bone becomes inflamed and causes severe pain and inflammation and swelling of the skin over the affected area. Prompt treatment with high doses of antibiotics is required and this condition may take several weeks to heal. If treatment fails, the condition may spread requiring surgical removal of all infected bone, followed by bone grafts and long-term antibiotic treatment.

Osteoporosis (OŚ-tē-ō-pō-RŌ-sis)

Osteoporosis is a common bone disease. It is the result of a reduction in the bone density that causes a weakening of the bone and increases the risk of fracture. The disease is characterised by low bone mass and structural deterioration of bone tissue. It is detected using a bone scan called bone densitometry.

Treatment includes hormone replacement therapy, selective oestrogen receptor moderator and bisphonate drugs. There are several causes including: lack of stress on the bone brought about by inactivity, deficiency of protein in the diet, deficiency of vitamin D, the reduced secretion of oestrogen in post-menopausal women, and disease or drugs including alcohol. It is often called the 'silent disease' because bone loss occurs without any symptoms.

Rickets and osteomalacia (oŚ-tē-ōma-LĀ-she-ah)

Rickets is the result of reduced mineral content in bony tissue. The bones become soft and are easily deformed. Clinical features in children are knock-knees or bow-legged lower limbs. In adults, where this occurs after fusion of the epiphyses and bone calcification fails, the disorder is called osteomalacia. The condition is associated with vitamin D deficiency or resistance, but may also be drug induced.

Scoliosis (skō-lē-Ō-sis)

Scoliosis describes a sidewards bend in the vertebral column. The deformity is usually in the thoracic region. Causes of the condition may be congenital, poor posture, differences in leg length (one leg shorter than the other), paralysis of muscles on one side of the vertebrae or chronic sciatica.

Spondylosis

Spondylosis is the term used when degenerative processes occur in the spine. During the process of ageing, the fluid content of the intervertebral discs diminishes causing the disc to become thinner (causing loss of height). This affects the shock-absorbing properties of the disc and causes instability of the spine. Inflammation of the joints will result and cause pain.

6 Joints

The different bones of the body are held in place by flexible connective tissue that forms joints. Joints occur at any place where two or more bones meet (articulate). Joints are divided into three groups.

Fibrous (fixed or immovable) joints

- These contain connective tissue with collagen fibres.

- They contain no space between the articulating joints and the synovial cavity (si-NŌ-vē-al).

- They permit little or no movement.

- Sutures uniting the bones of the skull are an example of fibrous joints.

*Types of joints:

(a) Fibrous

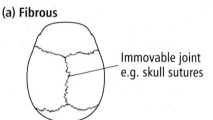

Immovable joint
e.g. skull sutures

Cartilaginous (kar-ti-LAJ-I-nus) joint

- These joints are fixed or slightly movable.

- There is no synovial cavity.

- Bones are held together with cartilage.

- This type of joint is found at the intervertebral joints between the bodies of the vertebrae and pubic symphysis.

(b) Cartilaginous

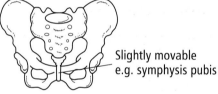

Slightly movable
e.g. symphysis pubis

Synovial joints (freely movable)

- These are freely movable.

- They have a synovial cavity to reduce friction of the joint during movement.

- The ends of the bone at a synovial joint are covered with smooth articular cartilage.

- The joint is enclosed in an articular capsule to unite the articulating bones.

- The articular capsule has two layers:

(c) Synovial

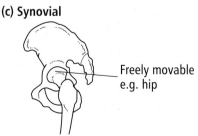

Freely movable
e.g. hip

* Diagrams to practise

- Fibrous capsule: the outer layer.
- Synovial membrane: the inner layer that secretes synovial fluid which lubricates, reduces friction, supplies nutrients and removes metabolic waste. It contains phagocytic cells that remove microbes and any debris created from normal wear of the joint.

- The fibrous capsule may contain bundles of fibres called ligaments, that are arranged in parallel bundles to help resist excess strain and prevent damage. Ligaments may lie inside or outside the articular capsule.

- Ligaments are tough fibrous bands containing elastin fibres that allow the ligament to stretch. Ligaments are attached to both ends of the articulating bone to help keep the two articular cartilages together.

- To reduce friction in joints that lie close to the skin, fluid-filled structures called bursae (BER-sē) cushion the movement. Bursae are filled with a fluid similar to synovial fluid and are present in the knee and shoulder joint.

Types of synovial joint

Synovial joints are classified into six sub-types, according to the range of movements they allow.

Types of synovial joint

Gliding (planar) joint   **Hinge joint**   **Pivot joint**

Condyloid joint   **Saddle joint**   **Ball and socket joint**

Planar joints

The articulating surfaces of bones are flat or slightly curved. Planar joints allow side to side and back and forth gliding movements.

Hinge joints

The articulating surfaces of the bones consist of one concave surface and one convex surface where one bone fits into the other. A hinge joint produces an open and close movement similar to the action of a hinge on a door.

Pivot joints

In this joint the end of one bone is rounded and the other has a ring or hole made of bone and ligament. A pivot joint allows rotational movement.

Condyloid joints (KON-di-loyd)

The articulating surface of one bone is an oval-shaped projection that fits into an oval-shaped depression of the other. This joint allows up and down and side to side movement.

Saddle joints

The articulating surface of one bone is saddle shaped with the articular surface of the other bone shaped to fit into the saddle. This type of joint allows side to side and up and down movement.

Ball and socket joints

In this joint a rounded ball-shaped surface fits into a cup-shaped depression that allows movement in several directions.

Knee joint

The knee joint is the largest joint in the body and it requires stabilising by ligaments and tendons. The knee joint is a hinge joint formed by the condyles of the femur and tibia and the posterior surface of the patella. The joint allows flexion and extension and a small degree of side to side movement when the knee is flexed. The joint has a joint capsule and extracapsular and intercapsular ligaments (cruciate ligaments) to strengthen it by limiting movement. The joint is further strengthened by two crescent wedge-shaped pieces of fibrous tissue called the menisci. The patella is a sesamoid bone that lies within the joint capsule. It slides on the patellar surface of the distal femur and its function is to reduce friction during extension and protect the knee joint.

Right knee joint

a) Front view

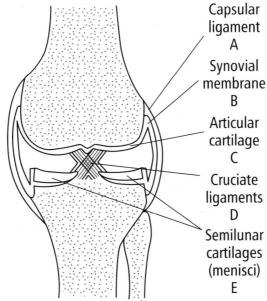

Capsular ligament
A

Synovial membrane
B

Articular cartilage
C

Cruciate ligaments
D

Semilunar cartilages (menisci)
E

A	=	Red
B	=	Light blue
C	=	Green
D	=	Orange
E	=	Purple
F	=	Pink
G	=	Dark blue
H	=	Brown
I	=	Yellow

b) Side view

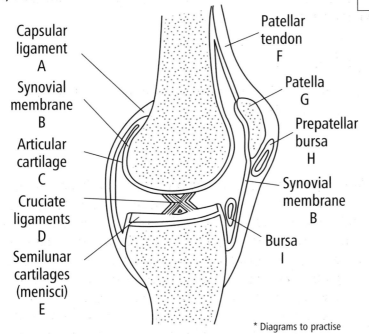

Capsular ligament
A

Synovial membrane
B

Articular cartilage
C

Cruciate ligaments
D

Semilunar cartilages (menisci)
E

Patellar tendon
F

Patella
G

Prepatellar bursa
H

Synovial membrane
B

Bursa
I

* Diagrams to practise

- Capsular ligament. Helps prevent dislocation. Stabilises joint.
- Synovial membrane. Secretes synovial fluid to lubricate and supply nutrients. Phagocytic cells are present to keep fluid free of debris.
- Articular cartilage. Reduces friction and acts as shock absorber.
- Cruciate ligaments. Strengthen and limit movement.
- Menisci. Fibrous tissue to ensure tight fit between joint surfaces of different shapes.
- Patella tendon. Helps prevent dislocation of patella. Stabilises joint.
- Patella. Sesamoid bone.
- Prepatella bursa. Sac of synovial fluid.
- Bursa. Sac of synovial fluid.

7 Types of movement

Synovial joints allow movement. The different sub-types of joint allow movement in specific planes. There are four main categories of joint movement:

Synovial joint movement

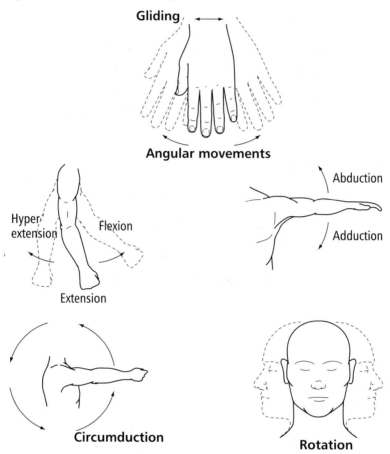

- Gliding.

- Angular movements: angular movements increase or decrease the angle between the articulating bones. There are four movements:
    - Flexion (FLEX-shun) causes a decrease in the angle by bending in.
    - Extension increases the angle by stretching out.
    - Abduction is the movement of bone away from the midline of the body.
    - Adduction is the movement towards the midline of the body.

- The circular motion allowed by ball and socket joints is called circumduction.

- Rotation: pivot and ball and socket joints allow a revolving movement.

Special movements

Specific joints are adapted to allow for special movements:

- Elevation and depression.

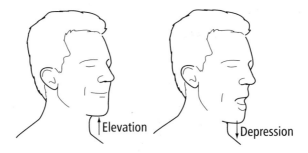

- Protraction and retraction.

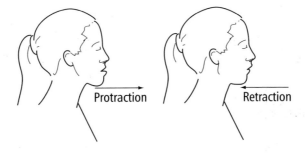

- Inversion and eversion.

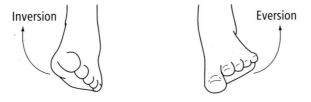

- Dorsiflexion and plantar flexion.
- Pronation and supination.

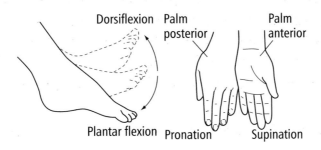

8 Diseases and disorders of joints

Gout

Gout develops when an abnormality of metabolism leads to an excess of uric acid in the blood. This produces crystals that are deposited in the soft tissue of the joints. The crystals cause irritation leading to inflammation, swelling and pain.

Osteoarthritis (os'-tē-ō-ar-THRĪ-tis)

Osteoarthritis is a degenerative joint disease that usually affects the large weight-bearing joints, mainly seen in people aged over 60. The articular cartilage is damaged and destroyed due to wear and tear, and early onset may be secondary to existing joint problems such as trauma. It is regarded as the leading cause of disability in older people. The loss of articular cartilage, development of bony spurs around the edges of the joint and thickening of the synovial membrane causes pain, swelling, stiffness and loss of joint function. Management includes anti-inflammatory drugs, pain relief using analgesia, physiotherapy, hydrotherapy and joint surgery to correct early deformities.

Rheumatism (ROO-ma-tism) and arthritis (ar-THRĪ-tis)

Rheumatism is the term used for any painful condition of the bones, ligaments, joints, tendons or muscle. Arthritis is the term used for rheumatism of the joints and it comes in many forms from a mild ache to severe pain with joint deformity. The cause of arthritis may be due to infection or problems associated with immunology, inflammation or degenerative conditions.

Rheumatoid arthritis (ROO-ma-toyd)

This is an autoimmune disease where the immune system attacks its own tissue. It causes a generalised inflammatory condition of connective tissue particularly in joints. Joint changes occur causing pain, swelling, severe deformity and loss of mobility. Management of rheumatoid arthritis may include joint-replacement therapy.

9 The muscular system

The skeleton and joints form the framework of the human body, but to produce movement components of muscle and tendons are needed.

Muscle is contractile tissue, designed to create movement of and within the body. Muscle tissue may constitute up to 50% of a person's body weight.

The movement or locomotor system is a complex series of coordinated functions of the skeletal, muscle and nervous system.

Function of muscle

- To create body movement.

- To stabilise body positions, for example keeping your head upright or enabling you to stand still or sit upright.

- To create heat: muscle movement creates heat to maintain normal body temperature.

- To act as a regulator for organs that allow the flow of fluid to and from temporary storage areas in hollow organs. For example the food in the stomach is able to be partially digested because of bands of muscle called sphincters. Sphincters prevent the contents of the stomach being vomited back out or from entering the intestines before partial digestion has taken place.

- To assist in moving substances, for example moving food and substances through the digestive system.

Types of muscle

Three types of muscle are found in the human body.

Voluntary or skeletal muscle

- Attached to the skeleton.

- Concerned with movement and locomotion.

- Activated by a conscious demand.

- When viewed under a microscope it has a striped appearance and is also known as striated muscle.

- It fatigues rapidly.

Skeletal muscle

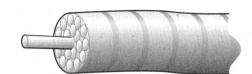

Smooth (involuntary or visceral) muscle

- This is found in the walls of hollow internal structures, i.e. arteries, veins and the intestines.

- It is regulated by the involuntary (autonomic) part of the nervous system, so a person has no control over the muscle contraction.

- Examined under a microscope the muscle has unstriated fibres that are arranged in bundles or sheets and is therefore also called smooth muscle.

- It fatigues slowly.

Distribution of smooth/involuntary muscle

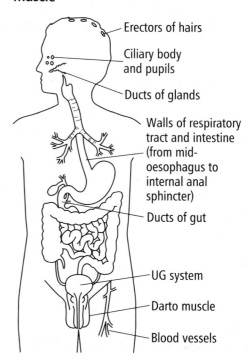

- Erectors of hairs
- Ciliary body and pupils
- Ducts of glands
- Walls of respiratory tract and intestine (from mid-oesophagus to internal anal sphincter)
- Ducts of gut
- UG system
- Darto muscle
- Blood vessels

Smooth muscle

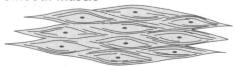

Cardiac muscle

- This is found only in the heart and at the cardiac ends of the main blood vessels.

- It is striated muscle but contractions are not under voluntary control.

- The special feature of cardiac muscle is its innate rhythmical activity.

- It contracts without fatigue.

Cardiac muscle

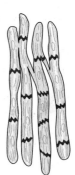

Elements required for function of muscles

There are four elements that are required for muscle tissue function:

- Excitability: it reacts to electrical signals from the nervous system.

- Contractibility: muscle tissue is able to become shorter and thicker (to contract).

- Extensibility: muscle tissue is able to stretch (extend) without causing damage.

- Elasticity: muscle tissue is able to go back to its original shape when relaxed.

Skeletal muscle

Most skeletal muscle lies just below the skin and there are approximately 600 named muscles in the body. Skeletal muscle is the only muscle tissue that may be controlled voluntarily, although in many cases this control operates through reflexes.

General anatomy and physiology of skeletal muscle

A whole muscle is made up of numerous muscle fibres and enclosed in a layer of connective tissue. Skeletal muscles are well supplied with nerves and blood vessels.

Skeletal muscle is stimulated by nerves of the peripheral nervous system and can produce rapid and forceful contractions needed for movement.

In most cases skeletal muscle has two ends that attach to other tissues and a wide middle section called the belly.

Muscle connects to bone by tendons. Tendons are tough strands or cords of fibrous tissue.

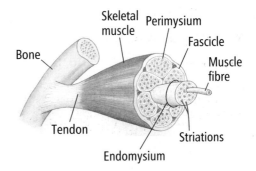

Gross structure of muscle

Bone, Skeletal muscle, Perimysium, Fascicle, Muscle fibre, Tendon, Striations, Endomysium

Structure of skeletal muscle

- The muscle is enclosed by a sheet of connective tissue – the deep fascia (FASH-ē-a)- that separates and holds muscles together.

- The outer covers of the muscle fibres also extend and form tendons that are the connective tissue that attaches the bone to the muscle.

- Under the deep fascia are bundles of muscle fibres called fascicles (FAS-I-kuls) that are covered by perimysium (per'-I-MĪZ-ē-um).

- Each individual muscle fibre is covered with endomysium (en' dō-MĪ Z-ē um).

- The muscle fibres contain a series of transverse strips of muscle protein, hence the name striped or striated muscle.

- Each muscle fibre is covered with a plasma membrane called sarcolemma from which extend small vessels called transverse tubules.

Muscle fibre

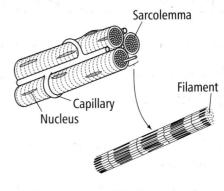

Sarcolemma, Nucleus, Capillary, Filament

Myofibril

- Sarcoplasm (the name for muscle cytoplasm) in each muscle fibre stores glycogen and oxygen (myoglobin) to provide energy during a muscle contraction.

- Along the length of each muscle fibre are tube-like structures called myofibrils.

- The myofibrils consist of interlinking thick and thin filaments.

- The thick myofibril filament is composed of a protein called myosin.

- The thin myofibril filament is composed of the protein called actin.

- The thick and thin filaments overlap in pattern and form the functional units of the muscle. The units are called sarcomers.

- Sarcomers are separated from each other by a zigzag band of dense material that is called the Z disc.

- Sarcomers have bands of filaments. The A band extends along the length of the thick filament and in its centre is a narrow band called the H zone. At each end of the A band, thick and thin filaments overlap. Thin filaments create the I band on either side of the A band. The I band is divided in half by a Z disc.

- One sarcomer is the region between two Z lines.

Sarcomer and filament

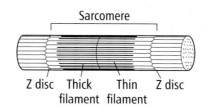

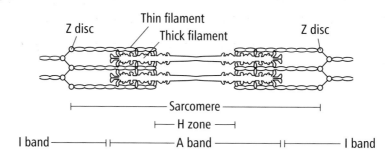

- The process of muscle contraction is stimulated by nerve impulses conducted via motor neurons. Neurons and muscle meet at the neuromuscular junction (NMJ). The NMJ provides a space/synapse across which messages from the impulse will travel.

Neuromuscular junction

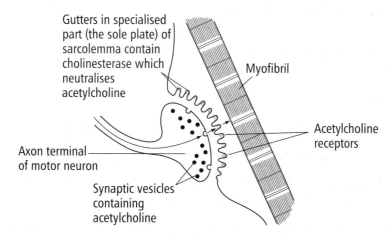

- At the axon terminal there are vesicles containing a neurotransmitter, i.e. Acetylcholine (ACh). When a nerve impulse is received the vesicle fuses with the cell membrane and released ACh.

- The ACh is moved across the synapse due to active transport promoted by high concentrations of sodium and potassium.

- The ACh attached to ACh receptors on the muscle cell membrane (sarcolemma) and this opens up a channel to allow the high concentration levels of sodium to flood into the cell.

- The change in sodium concentrations within the cell causes the sarcoplasmic reticula to release calcium.

- Calcium binds with the troponin molecules. This changes the shape of the troponin molecule and in turn the tropomyosin molecule, allowing the sliding filament mechanism of muscle contraction to take place.

- To relax the muscle, ACh is removed from the synaptic cleft by the action of Acetylcholinesterase (AChE).

10 The sliding-filament mechanism of muscle contraction

The troponin and tropomyosin molecules on the thin filament (actin) prevent contraction of the muscle. If calcium is released it changes the shape of these molecules to allow the myosin binding sites to be exposed. Heads on the thick filament (myosin) are able to bind with the actin and create crossbridges.

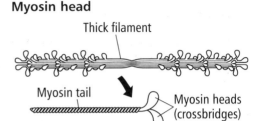

Myosin head

Thick filament

Myosin tail

Myosin heads (crossbridges)

The binding causes rigidity of the muscle and changes the shape of the molecules drawing the thin filament closer to the centre of the sacromere. Adenosine triphospate (ATP – an energy-carrying molecule manufactured in all living cells) is then required to break the crossbridge. The myosin head contains an enzyme, ATPhase which breaks down ATP into adenosine diphosphate (ADP). This action causes the myosin head to rotate before breaking the crossbridge, producing a power stroke that moves the thin filament closer to the centre allowing the myosin-binding site to bind with the next myosin head. The repeated formation and breaking of crossbridges requires a great deal of ATP. If ATP supplies are decreased, muscle fatigue will develop.

This will lead to a build-up of waste products, in particular lactic acid and carbon dioxide, and cause pain and stiffness in the affected muscles.

*Pattern of muscle contraction

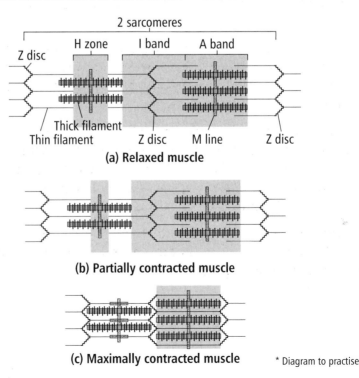

2 sarcomeres

Z disc · H zone · I band · A band · Thick filament · Thin filament · Z disc · M line · Z disc

(a) Relaxed muscle

(b) Partially contracted muscle

(c) Maximally contracted muscle

* Diagram to practise

The relaxation and contraction of muscle fibres has been studied under electron microscope. The pattern of movement is consistent.

In contracted muscle:

- A band remains unchanged.
- I band becomes shorter.
- H zone is not visible.

Relaxation of muscle occurs when the action potential stops and calcium moves back into the sarcoplasmic reticulum. This stops cross bridges being made.

Types of skeletal muscle contraction

Muscles contract to produce tension that will maintain the tone of the muscle or move the skeleton. The tension of the muscle must be able to produce a force that will be sufficient to produce the movement required. Picking up a pencil or a bag full of books will demand different tensions to overcome the weight of the two objects.

The muscle prepares for tension and contraction by producing a *twitch contraction* before the actual contraction begins. When the muscle fibres are stimulated to contract, a short spasmodic contraction followed by a period of relaxation occurs.

If the stimulus is repeated, the muscle continues spasmodic contractions that increase in intensity called *treppe*. Warm-up exercises before physical activity are aimed at producing treppe to prepare the muscle to produce maximum effort.

If the muscle is not allowed to relax due to repeated stimulation, the twitch contractions will produce a powerful continuous contraction called *tetany*. The powerful contraction reduces the oxygen supply to the muscle fibres and this causes pain.

Tetany may occur following physical activity and it is called cramp. Cramp may also occur with lower-level muscle activity after sitting awkwardly and this is then called a spasm. If tetany occurs there will be a period of intense pain until the muscle receives oxygen. Massage will help to speed up the return of the oxygen supply and relieve the pain.

Tension of the muscle is required to move an object. When the object is moving the muscle shortens as the skeletal joint moves. No further tension is required and this contraction is called isotonic.

When lifting a heavy object the tension of the muscle must be increased before the object can be moved. The muscle length stays the same although contraction is occurring. This contraction is called isometric.

When lifting objects, isotonic and isometric contractions are needed for movement.

Antagonist and prime mover

Shortening of the muscle, the tension remaining the same results in

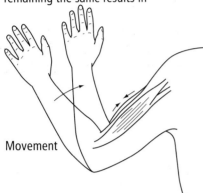

Movement

Increasing the tension, the length of the muscle remaining the same, results in:

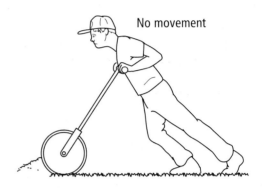

No movement

Muscle spindle

Allowing information from the muscle to be relayed back to the brain.

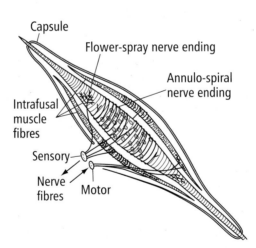

Capsule

Flower-spray nerve ending

Annulo-spiral nerve ending

Intrafusal muscle fibres

Sensory

Nerve fibres   Motor

- The brain is able to control muscle contraction by the number of motor units activated at one time.

- To transmit information from the muscle to the brain, the muscle fibres have tiny organs called muscle spindles that are connected to sensory nerves. The sensory nerve pathway is able to transmit continuous information to the brain to give feedback on the status of the muscle fibres.

- Muscles require a certain amount of contraction or tension to maintain muscle tone. Muscle tone keeps the muscle in a state of tension. Tension is needed in order to maintain posture.

Skeletal muscular system

Muscles may work independently or in coordination to allow smooth and precise movement. Muscles attached to a joint often work in pairs so that if one muscle contracts the other muscle will relax.

- Muscles that have the main responsibility for an action because they move and contract are called prime movers.

- Muscles that limit and counteract the movement are called antagonists. In a pair of working muscles the roles may be reversed.

- Groups of muscles that work together to produce a movement are called synergists. Synergists work to assist the prime mover and stabilise joints. Synergists may also prevent a movement at a joint, and the group of muscles is then called a fixator.

Muscle contraction

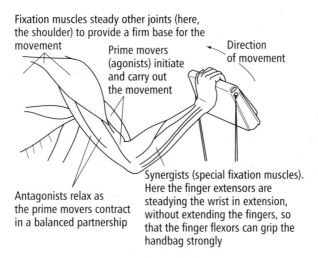

Fixation muscles steady other joints (here, the shoulder) to provide a firm base for the movement

Prime movers (agonists) initiate and carry out the movement

Direction of movement

Antagonists relax as the prime movers contract in a balanced partnership

Synergists (special fixation muscles). Here the finger extensors are steadying the wrist in extension, without extending the fingers, so that the finger flexors can grip the handbag strongly

The biceps are the prime mover to flex the elbow, and they are the antagonist when the elbow is lowered.

Information on the tension and state of the muscles is transmitted to the brain via receptors in the muscle called muscle spindles. The muscle spindle is a collection of modified muscle fibres that are enclosed in connective tissue. The connective tissue connects the receptor to surrounding muscle fibres. As the muscle fibres move, the spindle becomes elongated and information about muscle activity is transmitted to the brain. Similar receptors are also present in the tendons.

Principal muscles

The name of muscles often relates to their size, position, function and shape. As previously stated there are over 600 muscles in the body and it is not necessary at this stage to remember details about all of them.

The following diagrams illustrate the position and names of muscles that are relevant to understanding the principles of movement and posture relating to healthcare.

Muscles of the body: anterior view

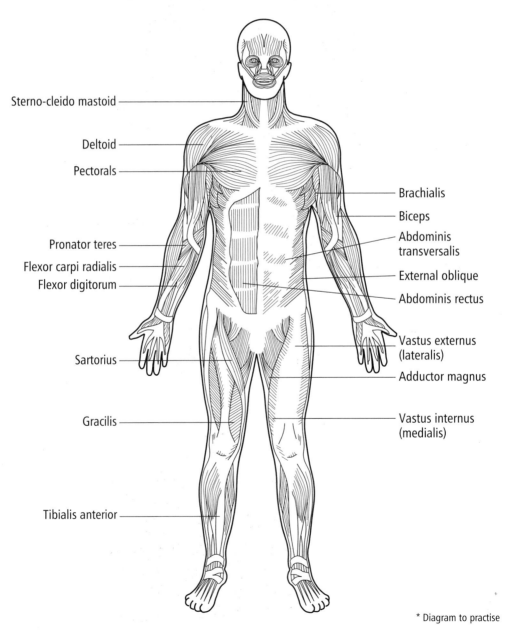

Sterno-cleido mastoid

Deltoid

Pectorals

Brachialis

Biceps

Abdominis transversalis

Pronator teres

Flexor carpi radialis

External oblique

Flexor digitorum

Abdominis rectus

Vastus externus (lateralis)

Sartorius

Adductor magnus

Gracilis

Vastus internus (medialis)

Tibialis anterior

* Diagram to practise

Muscles of the body: posterior view

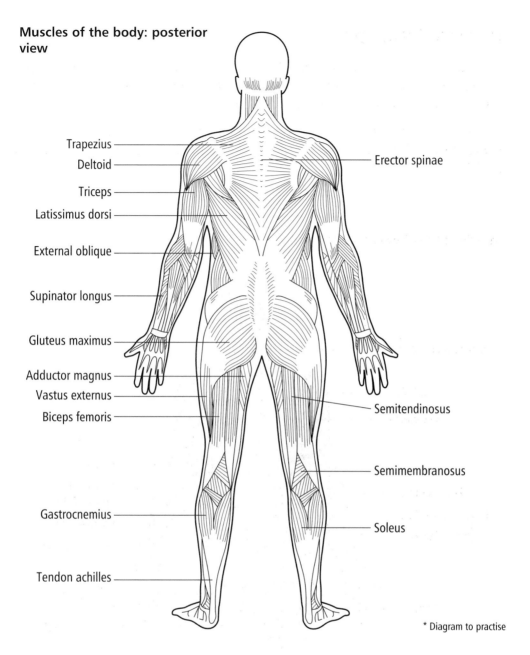

Trapezius

Deltoid

Triceps

Latissimus dorsi

External oblique

Supinator longus

Gluteus maximus

Adductor magnus

Vastus externus

Biceps femoris

Gastrocnemius

Tendon achilles

Erector spinae

Semitendinosus

Semimembranosus

Soleus

* Diagram to practise

Muscles of the head and neck

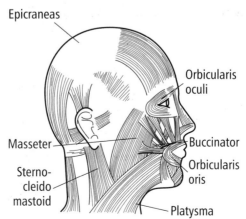

Epicraneas

Orbicularis oculi

Masseter

Buccinator

Sterno-cleido mastoid

Orbicularis oris

Platysma

Superficial muscles of the forearms

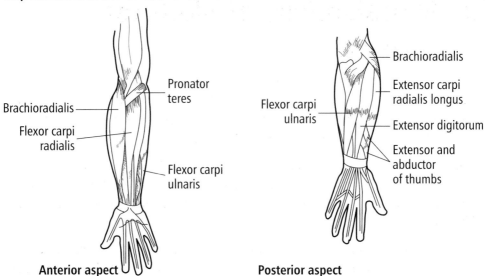

Brachioradialis

Pronator teres

Flexor carpi radialis

Flexor carpi ulnaris

Anterior aspect

Brachioradialis

Extensor carpi radialis longus

Flexor carpi ulnaris

Extensor digitorum

Extensor and abductor of thumbs

Posterior aspect

Posterior and anterior views of muscles of the leg

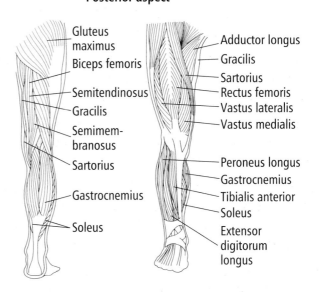

Gluteus maximus

Biceps femoris

Semitendinosus

Gracilis

Semimembranosus

Sartorius

Gastrocnemius

Soleus

Adductor longus

Gracilis

Sartorius

Rectus femoris

Vastus lateralis

Vastus medialis

Peroneus longus

Gastrocnemius

Tibialis anterior

Soleus

Extensor digitorum longus

Superficial muscles of the lower leg

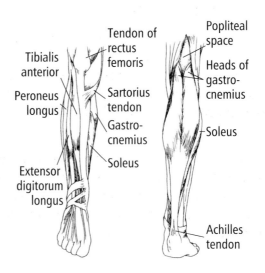

Tibialis anterior

Peroneus longus

Extensor digitorum longus

Tendon of rectus femoris

Sartorius tendon

Gastrocnemius

Soleus

Popliteal space

Heads of gastrocnemius

Soleus

Achilles tendon

11 Metabolism of skeletal muscle

Adenosine triphosphate (ATP) is the immediate source of energy for muscle contraction. Muscle fibres contain enough ATP to power the inactive muscle for a few seconds of strenuous activity. If the activity continues, more ATP is required. Muscle fibres get additional ATP from three sources:

- Creatine phosphate: an energy-rich molecule. It derives its energy from a phosphate from ATP and then transfers the energy to ADP to make more ATP. This provides sufficient energy for short bursts of activity lasting up to 15 seconds.

- Glucogen: when the supply of creatine phosphate has been depleted, the muscle fibre uses glucose from its store and the blood. The breakdown of glucogen molecules produces ATP and lactic acid. This provides energy for a period of approximately 30 seconds.

- Aerobic cellular respiration: muscle fibres are able to receive oxygen from the blood and the myoglobin in sarcoplasm. Myoglobin releases oxygen that generates ATP from glucose molecules.

During the oxidation of glycogen pyruvic acid is formed. If oxygen is available pyruvic acid is broken down to carbon dioxide and water and during this process energy is released producing more ATP.

If there is insufficient oxygen, the pyruvic acid is converted to lactic acid. Lactic acid is transported in the blood to the liver where it is converted back to glucose. The presence of lactic acid in the blood stimulates the respiratory centre and the rate and depth of respiration is increased.

The muscle will continue to receive energy until the level of calcium drops and there are insufficient supplies of creatine phosphate, glucogen and oxygen to cope with the build-up of lactic acid.

Increased respiration rate continues immediately after exercise has stopped until sufficient oxygen has been transported around the body to oxidise the lactic acid or convert it to glycogen. The extra oxygen needed to convert lactic acid to glucogen, replace oxygen in myoglobin and reform creatine phosphate and ATP is called oxygen debt. The oxygen debt must be replenished after exercise.

If, as a result of immobility, muscle fibres are not used, the muscle bulk will decrease and be replaced by fibrous tissue. This will result in muscle weakness and a reduction in mobility. Therefore, it is very important to encourage clients with mobility problems to participate in passive or active physiotherapy exercises to prevent muscle wasting.

12 Diseases and disorders of muscles

Abnormal contractions of skeletal muscle

- Cramp: this is a painful muscle contraction that may occur after exercise or in the legs at night. It is not usually a symptom of disease.

- Spasm: a sudden abnormal muscle contraction of a single muscle that belongs to a large group of muscles.

- Tremor: a rhythmic movement of parts of the body that is involuntary. The rhythmic contraction of the muscles produces a quivering or shaking movement.

Back pain

Low back pain is a very common problem in industrialised society. In most cases pain originates in the invertebral joints and back muscles. The back muscles are the antagonists of the abdominal muscles and additional work is necessary to support the abdominal muscles during pregnancy or if a person is obese. Pain may also arise from trauma to the muscles following physical exertion or the lifting of heavy objects.

Muscular dystrophy

Muscular dystrophy relates to an inherited group of disorders causing degeneration of individual muscle fibres leading to a progressive wasting of skeletal muscle.

Myasthenia gravis (mī-as-THĒ-nē-a GRAV-is)

This condition is a chronic and progressive neuromuscular disease that develops in early adulthood. The muscle acetylcholine receptors are blocked by antibodies and as the disease progresses muscles become permanently weakened. This condition is more common in women. Muscle groups commonly affected are the face, neck and limbs. Initial symptoms include drooping of the eyelid, double vision due to eye muscle weakness and difficulty in swallowing.

Further reading

Cree, L. and Rischmiller, S. (1991) *Science in Nursing*, 2nd edn. Baillière Tindall, Sydney.

Ford, S. and Richards, A. (1995) *Human Physiology and Health in the Care Context*. Nelson Thornes, Cheltenham.

Klippel, J. and Dieppe, P. A. (1994) *Rheumatology*. Mosby, London.

Memmler, R. L. and Cohen, B. J. (1996) *Structure and Function of the Human Body*. J. B. Lippincott, Philadelphia.

Chapter 3
The cardiovascular system

National unit specification
These are the topics you will be studying for this unit.

1   The cardiovascular system

2   Location, function and anatomy of the heart

3   The cardiac cycle

4   Conduction system of the heart and methods of recording heart activity

5   Diseases and disorders of the heart

6   The circulatory system

7   Functions and composition of blood

8   Blood groups and rhesus factors

9   Diseases and disorders of the circulatory system and blood

---

Diagrams to practise:

Cardiovascular system

Structure of the heart

Blood flow through the heart during systole and diastole

Anatomy of arteries and veins

Your learning outcomes may include demonstrating knowledge of the basic anatomy and functions of the cardiovascular system and assessments in the form of a time-constraint test. You may also have to present experiments in the form of written reports.

Homeostasis

The cardiovascular system delivers oxygen and nutrients to all cells in the body and removes waste.

Skin:
Injury to skin is repaired by components of blood.
Blood is cooled or warmed as it flows through the layers of skin.

Skeleton:
Blood transports hormones, calcium and phosphate for bone development.

Muscle:
Blood removes waste products and heat from muscle after exercise.

Nervous system:
Produces cerebrospinal fluid.

Endocrine system:
Blood transports hormones to target cells.

Lymph:
Carries cells to help immune system and forms interstitial fluid.

Respiratory system:
Transports oxygen and carbon dioxide.

Digestive system:
Transports nutrients and hormones.

Urinary system:
Filters blood and uses unwanted water and substances to produce urine.

Reproductive system:
Distributes hormones.
Vasodilation causes erection of penis and clitoris.

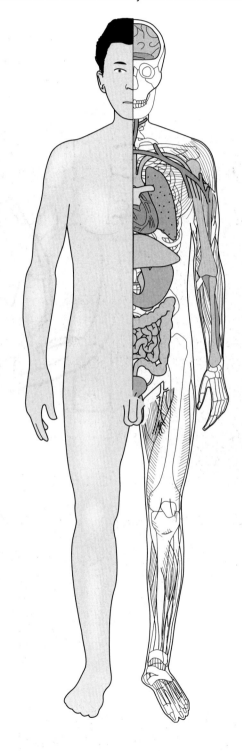

1 The cardiovascular system

The cardiovascular system is a system of vessels that transports blood and circulatory fluids to and from all areas of the body. In the human body this is a closed system that consists of:

- Heart: a 'pumping' organ.

- Blood vessels: a closed circuit of tubes.

- Arteries: carry blood to all parts of the body.

- Capillaries: leak fluid out to body cells and collect waste.

- Veins: carry blood back to the heart.

- Blood: consisting mainly of the liquid plasma.

Circulatory system

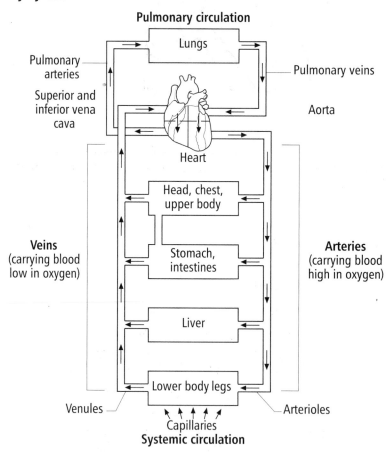

In our bodies blood flows through approximately 96 500 kilometres of arteries and veins. The circulatory system plays a vital role in the process of various body functions including respiration, nutrition and the removal of waste products.

2 Location, function and anatomy of the heart

The heart is a muscular organ that is situated in the chest cavity between the lungs just under the sternum and above the diaphragm, in a space called the mediastinum.

Position of the heart

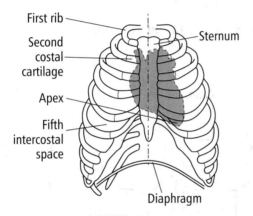

The human heart is conical in shape with flattened back and front surfaces. In a healthy person the heart is the size of their closed fist. However, it varies in size according to the person's age, sex and weight.

Heart and associated blood vessels

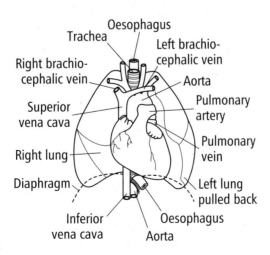

Anatomy of the heart

The heart consists of three layers: the pericardium, the myocardium and the endocardium.

The layers of the heart

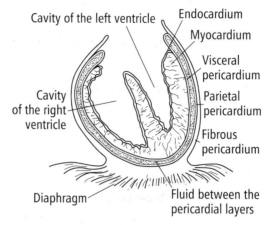

Cavity of the left ventricle

Endocardium

Myocardium

Visceral pericardium

Parietal pericardium

Fibrous pericardium

Cavity of the right ventricle

Diaphragm

Fluid between the pericardial layers

Pericardium

The heart is enclosed in a strong, protective membrane called the pericardium. The pericardium consists of a number of layers:

- Fibrous pericardium: connective tissue attached to the diaphragm and sternum.

- Parietal pericardium: connected to the fibrous pericardium.

- Visceral pericardium: connected to the myocardium.

There is a layer of fatty fluid between the parietal and visceral pericardium to hold the two layers together and prevent friction between the membranes when the heart beats (contracts).

Myocardium

Cardiac muscle

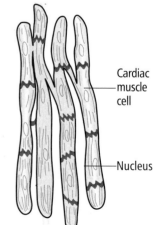

The myocardium contains cardiac muscle and forms the bulk of the heart wall. Cardiac muscle tissue contains striations of protein fibres in the muscle cells. The cells are stacked in columns and are connected by intercalated discs and branching muscle fibre that enable the cells to communicate with each other so that they all contract at the same time.

Cardiac muscle cell

Nucleus

Endocardium

The endocardium consists of endothelial tissue that lines the internal surface of the heart chambers and valves. In a healthy heart this tissue is smooth to allow blood to flow smoothly through the four chambers and vessels that join the heart.

Functions of the heart

- Circulates oxygenated blood to body tissues. The blood enters the systemic (high-pressure) circulation structures.

- Pumps deoxygenated blood to the lungs through the pulmonary (low-pressure) circulation.

The heart must maintain constant circulation of blood throughout the body to maintain homeostasis.

The pumping action of the heart and the flow of blood through and out of the heart is called the cardiac cycle.

The circulation of blood

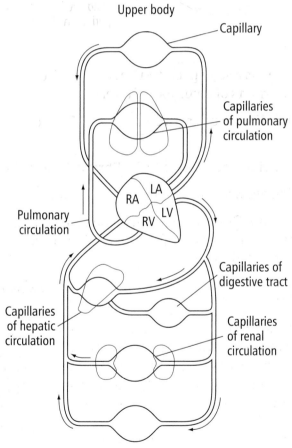

Upper body

Capillary

Capillaries of pulmonary circulation

RA · LA · LV · RV

Pulmonary circulation

Capillaries of digestive tract

Capillaries of hepatic circulation

Capillaries of renal circulation

Capillaries of lower limbs and body

* Diagram to practise

| Red | = | Circulation entering and leaving left side of heart |
| Blue | = | Circulation entering and leaving right side of heart |

Flow of blood through the heart

Internal structure of the heart and associated blood vessels

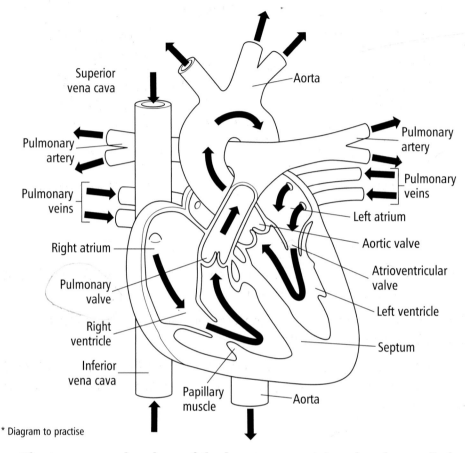

Labels: Superior vena cava, Aorta, Pulmonary artery, Pulmonary artery, Pulmonary veins, Pulmonary veins, Left atrium, Right atrium, Aortic valve, Atrioventricular valve, Pulmonary valve, Left ventricle, Right ventricle, Septum, Inferior vena cava, Papillary muscle, Aorta

* Diagram to practise

- The two upper chambers of the heart are receiving chambers called atria. (atria (plural), atrium (singular)).

- The two lower chambers that pump blood into the circulation are called ventricles.

- The two sides of the heart are divided by a septum.

- The two chambers on each side of the heart are separated by valves made of epithelial tissue that control blood flow.

- Heart valves allow blood flow in one direction only:
  - The atrioventricular valve (AV), between the atria and ventricles stops the backflow of blood when the ventricles contract. The atrioventricular valve between the left atrium and left ventricle is called the bicuspid or mitral valve. The AV valve between the right atria and ventricles is called the tricuspid valve. The opening and closing of the AV valves is due to pressure differences. When the blood flows from the atrium to the ventricle the valve is pushed open. Then, as the ventricle contracts, the blood pushes the cusps upward which closes the opening.

Atrioventricular valve

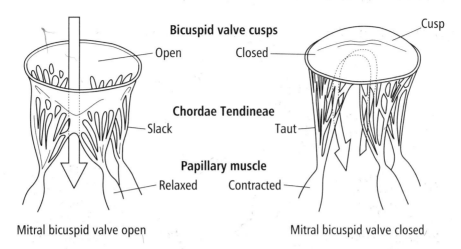

Bicuspid valve cusps
Open   Closed   Cusp

Chordae Tendineae
Slack   Taut

Papillary muscle
Relaxed   Contracted

Mitral bicuspid valve open   Mitral bicuspid valve closed

- Mitral valve/bicuspid valve: situated between the left ventricle and the left atrium which has two flaps or cusps.

- Tricuspid valve: situated between the right ventricle and the right atrium which has three flaps or cusps.

- Two halfmoon shaped (semilunar) valves are found at the entry points of the main blood vessels. These valves are shaped like pockets and open in one direction only.

Semilunar valve

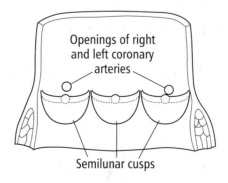

Openings of right and left coronary arteries

Semilunar cusps

- The 'lubb dub' heart sounds heard through a stethoscope are made when the valves of the heart close. The closing of the AV valves create the 'lubb', the first heart sound, and after a very short interval the semilunar valves close creating the 'dub' sound.

3 The cardiac cycle

The cardiac cycle is the term used for each heart beat. A heart beat consists of three different stages: diastole, atrial systole and ventricular systole.

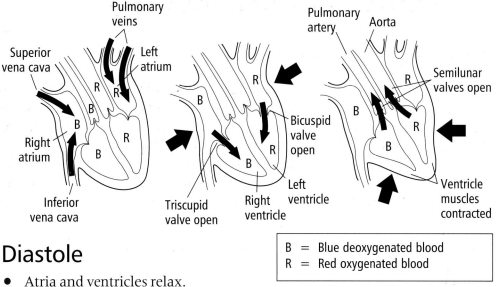

| B | = | Blue deoxygenated blood |
| R | = | Red oxygenated blood |

Diastole

- Atria and ventricles relax.
- Blood enters the heart, pulmonary veins and inferior vena cava.

Atrial systole

Both atria contract resulting in a decrease of volume. This increases the blood pressure within the atria, allowing blood to flow at high pressure through the tricuspid and bicuspid valves into the ventricles.

Ventricular systole

Both ventricles contract and the atria begins to relax. As the ventricles contract and volume decreases so the pressure increases. When the pressure in the ventricles is greater than in the atria, the tricuspid and bicuspid valves will be closed. When the pressure in the ventricles is greater than that of the arteries, the semilunar valve will be pushed open to allow the blood to flow through to the aorta and pulmonary arteries.

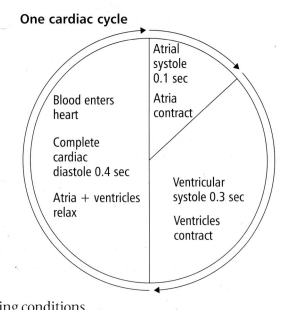

The contraction and relaxation cycle is repeated 70–80 times a minute in a healthy heart under resting conditions.

4 Conduction system of the heart and methods of recording heart activity

Conduction system

The heart muscle is prompted to relax and constrict by an internal electrical system that is able to work independently of the nervous system. The coordinated contraction of the heart is made possible because of the specialised cardiac muscle cells and the structure of the myocardium. An internal control centre or pacemaker, called the sinoatrial node, controls the beating of the heart with additional input from the autonomic nervous system. During an average lifetime, the heart beats more than 2000 million times.

Conduction of the heart beat and pathways of conduction

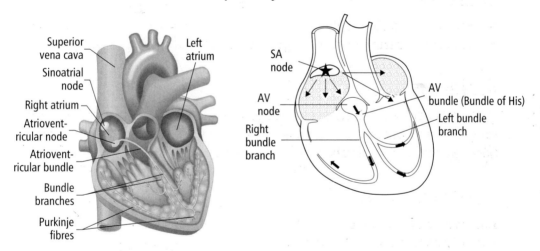

- Impulses are discharged from the sinoatrial (SA) node (also called a pacemaker).

- The SA node contains special cells which are regulated by the nervous and endocrine system.

- The impulse spreads throughout the muscle of both atria, which are 'excited' and contract.

- This impulse is passed to the atrioventricular (AV) node that is situated in the right atrium next to the tricuspid valve. Conduction is delayed momentarily at the AV node to allow the atria time to empty blood into the ventricles.

- The electrical impulse then passes down a structure called the atrioventricular bundle (Bundle of His).

- The impulse is relayed by the Purkinje fibres to the ventricular muscle cells which cause them to contract simultaneously creating a coordinated ventricular systole action.

Measuring activity

The wave of excitement spreading through the heart muscle is accompanied by electrical charges that are conducted to the surface of the body. The electrical events may be recorded using monitoring equipment called an electrocardiogram (ECG).

Electrocardiogram

Taking an ECG

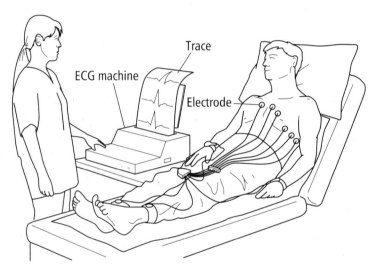

Electrodes are placed on the chest wall and the arms and legs of the client. The ECG is then displayed as a paper tracing or graphically on an oscilloscope. A healthy heart will produce a typical waveform with peaks and troughs in the recording that show changes in the electrical events during one beat of the heart. A typical ECG will show a waveform of sinus

Normal electrocardiograph tracing

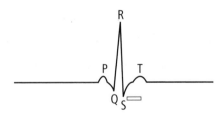

Time = 0.8 seconds

rhythm with deflective waves known as the PQRST complex. Alterations from typical waveforms and sinus rhythm may indicate problems with the conductive system or cardiac muscle. The ECG is a useful diagnostic aid to identify heart disease or disorders.

- Time = 0.8 seconds.
- P wave = shows the electrical activity that progresses through the atria.
- QRS waves = the changes in the electrical activity that progresses through the ventricles.
- T wave = diastole: ventricles relaxed.

Cardiac output

- The volume of blood pumped out of the ventricles in each minute is called the cardiac output (CO).
- The CO depends on the heart rate (HR) and stroke volume (SV).
- Stroke volume is the amount of blood pumped out during ventricular contractions.
- Cardiac output is a factor important in the maintenance of normal blood pressure.

Heart rate

The average adult heart rate is 60–80 beats per minute. The heart rate will vary in response to the needs of the body. The heart rate depends on the activity of the sinoatrial node that is controlled by the vagus nerve (which slows the rate) and the sympathetic nerves (which increase the rate). If damage occurs to the sinoatrial node the atrioventricular node takes over the function as it is unaffected by external influences. This node has its own contraction rate of 35–45 beats per minute.

- When a person is resting, if the rate is over 100 beats a minute it is termed tachycardia.
- When a person is resting, if the rate is below 60 beats a minute it is termed bradycardia.
- The cardiovascular centre (CVC) controls the rate and force of each heart beat. The CVC is situated in the medulla area of the brain.
- The vasomotor centre controls blood vessel size and blood pressure.

Regulation of heart beat

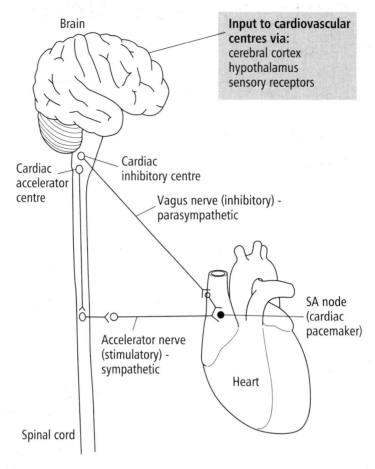

Blood supply to the heart

The heart is supplied with arterial (oxygenated) blood by the right and left coronary arteries that originate from the aorta. The arteries divide up into a network of smaller arteries that enclose the heart in a crown-like pattern. The venous (deoxygenated) blood drains into the coronary veins taking the blood directly back to the right atrium. Blood supply takes place while the heart is in diastole and the heart receives approximately 250 ml of blood per minute.

5 Diseases and disorders of the heart

Abnormal cardiac function

Acute circulatory failure

This is when the cardiac output is not sufficient to maintain blood pressure and therefore perfusion of all body tissue is compromised. The various causes of acute circulatory failure include:

- Hypovolemia: a decrease in blood volume caused by factors including haemorrhage, loss of body fluids through vomiting and diarrhoea.

- Cardiogenic: the heart failing to pump due to muscle damage.

- Vascular: where the body responds to shock, causing a reduction in the circulating blood volume.

Heart failure

Heart failure occurs when the heart cannot maintain sufficient circulation to meet the body's current circulatory requirements. If the output of the heart is reduced but blood still returns with the same or increased filling pressure, there will be congestion and a backlog of blood waiting to enter into the heart. When the venous pressure is increased and there is pulmonary and peripheral congestion it is called congestive cardiac failure.

Coronary heart disease (CHD)

Coronary heart disease is a major medical, social and economic hazard in industrialised countries. The Department of Health issued statistical data stating that the number of deaths due to CHD in the UK were among the highest in western Europe. Health policies to date have attempted to address issues relating to CHD by promoting healthy eating and healthy lifestyles and establishing improved coronary care facilities. (*Saving Lives: Our Healthier Nation*, 1999)

Any interruption to the homeostatic control of the cardiac function will have a severe effect on the heart cells and their function. Examples of CHD are:

Angina pectoris

Angina pectoris is pain in the chest, neck and right arm caused by a gradual build-up of atheroma within the coronary arteries. Atheroma is an abnormal mass of fatty or lipid material deposited in an arterial wall. The heart will not receive sufficient oxygen during stressful conditions or physical exertion.

Coronary atherosclerosis

A disease developed when fatty lesions form below the endothelial lining of the coronary arteries. This may lead to hardening, narrowing and possible blockage (occlusion) of the artery.

Coronary artery disease

This term refers to the clinical manifestations of coronary atherosclerosis. A person may have coronary atherosclerosis without exhibiting clinical signs, resulting in an unexpected sudden death.

Coronary occlusion

When a thrombosis occurs it may obstruct the flow of blood through a coronary artery. The obstruction may be caused by bleeding (haemorrhage) below the endothelial lining, or from an embolus. An embolus is a clot that is formed elsewhere and passes through the vessels into the coronary arteries.

Coronary thrombosis

A clot (thrombus) forms in the coronary arterial system, usually in relation to an abnormality of the lining of the artery.

Myocardial infarction (MI)

A myocardial infarction (heart attack or coronary) is the death of part of the cardiac muscle following interruption of its blood supply due to coronary thrombosis or occlusion.

6 The circulatory system

The heart and blood vessels within the body form a completely closed circuit. Humans have double circulation whereby each red blood cell passes through the heart twice. The circulatory system is divided into two systems:

- Systemic circulation: the flow of blood around the body.

- Pulmonary circulation: the flow of blood to and from the lungs.

The blood vessels are the transport system for the blood which delivers energy and food to all cells in the body and removes waste products. There are three basic types of vessels: arteries, capillaries and veins.

Arteries

Arteries carry blood away from the heart. With the exception of the pulmonary artery, the blood is oxygenated. The size of arteries throughout the body varies. There are large elastic arteries that conduct the blood away from the heart, medium-size muscular arteries that distribute the blood around the body and tiny arterioles that join the capillaries.

Arterial tree

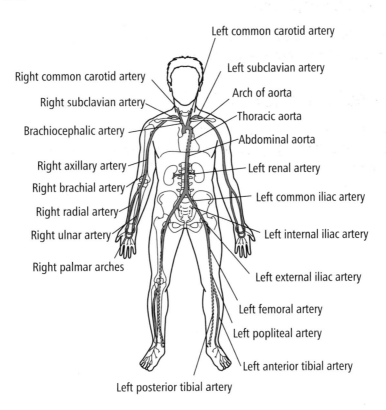

Left common carotid artery

Right common carotid artery

Left subclavian artery

Right subclavian artery

Arch of aorta

Brachiocephalic artery

Thoracic aorta

Abdominal aorta

Right axillary artery

Left renal artery

Right brachial artery

Left common iliac artery

Right radial artery

Right ulnar artery

Left internal iliac artery

Right palmar arches

Left external iliac artery

Left femoral artery

Left popliteal artery

Left anterior tibial artery

Left posterior tibial artery

Arteries are constructed of three layers of tissue plus layers of elastic fibres called elastic lamina:

Coronary artery

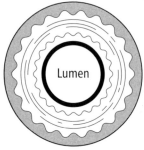

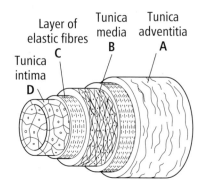

A =	Green
B =	Orange
C =	Light blue
D =	Pink

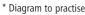

* Diagram to practise

- Outer layer: the tunica adventitia layer that consists of fibrous connective tissue.

- Middle layer: the tunica media layer that consists of smooth muscle and elastic tissue. The smooth muscle contains sympathetic nerve fibres. When the muscle contracts the diameter of the artery is reduced causing vasoconstriction.

- Internal layer: the tunica intima layer that consists of squamous epithelia called the endothelium. The epithelial cells are flat to ensure the internal lining of the artery is smooth and does not impede the flow of blood.

Pulse

The arteries share the function of blood-pressure regulators. The elastic tissue of the artery stretches as blood is pumped through and limits the systolic arterial blood pressure. During diastole the elastic fibres recoil, returning the energy stored in the vessel wall to the blood. The pulsating movement of the artery walls due to the change in arterial pressure is the basis of the pulse. The pulse is best recorded in specific locations where the arteries pass close to the skin. The number of pulses felt in one minute is recorded as the heart rate. Pulse rates vary as a result of age, posture, temperature and level of fitness. The rhythm and strength of the pulse should be a

Locations for taking a pulse

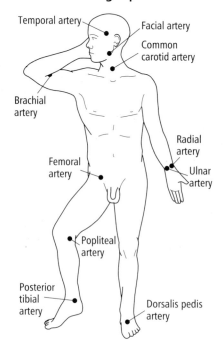

regular pattern. A very fast pulse (tachycardia) or very slow pulse (bradycardia) will result in inadequate filling of the coronary arteries.

1. Use two fingers to locate your radial pulse as shown in the diagram.

2. If you cannot feel the pulse, slightly change the position or increase the pressure of your fingertips.

3. Note the rate, rhythm and strength of the pulse.

Taking a radial pulse

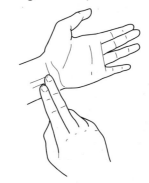

Blood pressure

As oxygenated blood is discharged from the left ventricle, the force or pressure that the blood exerts on the artery walls is known as systolic blood pressure. When the heart rests (cardiac diastole), the pressure in the artery falls to give a diastolic blood pressure.

Blood pressure (BP) is measured using a millimetre of mercury (Hg) or in kilopascals (kPa) as units of pressure. In a healthy young adult, systolic blood pressure should be 90–120mm Hg and diastolic pressure 60–90mm Hg (5 mm Hg = 0.66 kPa).

Blood pressure is measured using electronic measuring equipment and is usually recorded with the systolic pressure over the diastolic pressure: BP = 120/80mm Hg or 16/11 kPa.

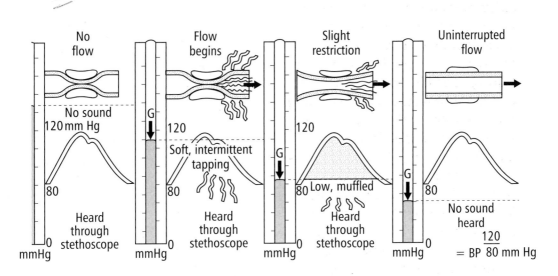

Digital machines have now replaced the traditional mercury sphygmo-manometers. The pressure cuff is placed around the upper arm with a pressure pad over the brachial artery. The cuff will inflate until no pulse is felt and then slowly deflate. The first pulse felt is the systolic reading. The diastolic reading is when the pulse fades and is no longer detectable. Blood pressure is often recorded using the brachial artery of the arm.

Readings will vary depending on the position of the person (for example if they are sitting, standing or lying down), the age and gender.

Blood pressure will alter in order to maintain homeostasis. Factors that affect blood pressure are:

- Cardiac output: the rate and force of blood ejected from the heart.

- Blood volume: the amount of blood circulating throughout the body.

- Peripheral resistance: the thickness of blood (viscosity) is altered by the amount of red blood cells in the plasma. Additional red blood cells increase the amount of friction that blood encounters as it flows through the circulatory system. Resistance of the blood flow increases if blood vessels dilate to take additional blood to active organs in need of extra oxygen supplies. This causes low blood pressure.

- Elasticity of arterial walls: the elastic fibres help to push the blood through the arterial system.

- Venous return: the blood returning to the heart depends on gravity, muscular contraction, respiratory movement and the force of contractions of the left ventricle.

Capillaries

The small arteries, arterioles, become minute vessels called capillaries. The thin wall of a capillary is composed of a single layer of epithelial cells that allows an exchange of substances between the blood and tissues. Blood cells and plasma proteins have a large molecular substance and do not usually pass through the capillary wall. When it is necessary for larger molecules to permeate, the capillaries will have pores or a sinusoid channel to allow movement of hormones, proteins and sometimes blood vessels between the capillary and the cells. This is necessary in organs such as the kidney and liver.

Structure of a capillary

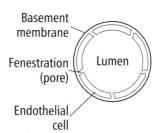

Basement membrane

Fenestration (pore)

Lumen

Endothelial cell

Capillary exchange

Blood flows slowly through the capillaries to allow the exchange of nutrients and waste between the cells and the blood. The exchange between the cells is made possible by diffusion (hydrostatic pressure) and bulk flow (osmotic colloid pressure).

Capillaries

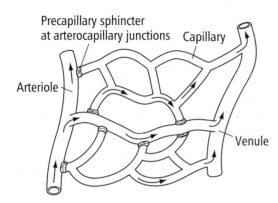

Precapillary sphincter at arterocapillary junctions   Capillary

Arteriole

Venule

Capillary exchange of gases

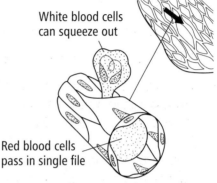

White blood cells can squeeze out

Red blood cells pass in single file

Hydrostatic pressure

The oxygen carried in the blood is exchanged between the arterial end of the capillaries and the tissue fluid. This occurs through a process called diffusion. The higher concentration of oxygen in the blood diffuses to a lower concentration in the tissues. Carbon dioxide, a waste product of the cells, diffuses into the blood towards the venous end of the capillary.

The effect of hydrostatic pressure

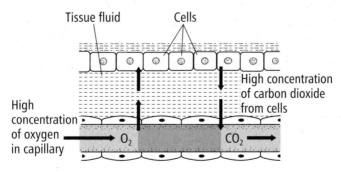

Tissue fluid   Cells

High concentration of carbon dioxide from cells

High concentration of oxygen in capillary → O_2

CO_2 →

Osmotic colloid pressure

Osmotic pressure

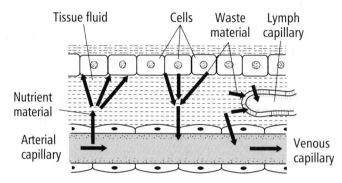

- Osmotic pressure is the pressure of a fluid. The pressure is caused by the solution of particles in the fluid, called solute concentration.

- The filtration of nutrients occurs as the pressure of blood against the wall of the capillary pushes fluid out of the capillary into interstitial fluid.

- The pressure in the capillary is higher than the blood colloid (surrounding tissue) causing the water, oxygen and solutes to move into the surrounding interstitial tissue – a passive process by which the solute concentrates move together, called bulk flow.

- The capillary blood pressure decreases as the blood flows through the capillary and will, about halfway along, be lower than the blood colloid osmotic pressure. The water and solubles in the interstitial fluid will then begin to bulk flow into the blood capillary for reabsorption.

- The reabsorbed fluid will contain carbon dioxide and other waste products.

Venules and veins

Structure of a vein

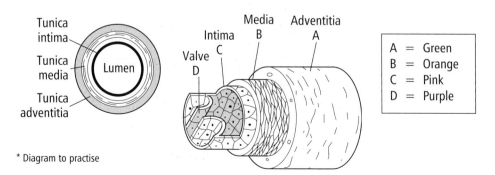

A =	Green
B =	Orange
C =	Pink
D =	Purple

* Diagram to practise

Veins carry blood to the heart. With the exception of the pulmonary veins the blood is deoxygenated – carrying waste carbon dioxide.

- Blood enters capillaries from arterioles.

- The capillaries connect to little veins called venules. Venules join to form small then larger veins.

- The flow of blood through veins will be slower than through arteries due to loss of pressure. Veins do not pulsate and the adjustment of capacity and regulation of blood flow back to the heart is controlled by modified smooth muscle.

Valves

Valves in a vein

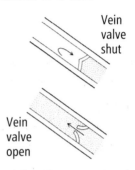

Vein valve shut

Vein valve open

- Veins have a similar structure to arteries, but they have a thinner inner and middle layer. The veins situated in the legs and arms have small valves made from folds of internal endothelium which prevent the blood flowing backwards.

- If the valves are weak gravity may force blood back through the valve, increasing the venous blood pressure and causing the vein wall to be

Venous tree

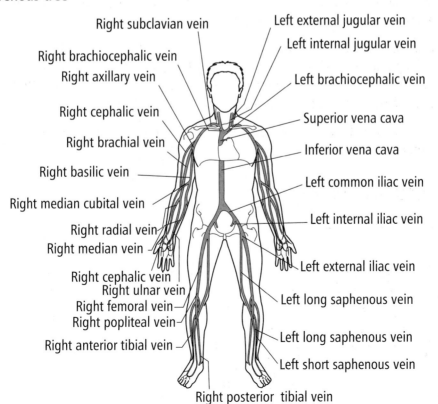

Right subclavian vein
Right brachiocephalic vein
Right axillary vein
Right cephalic vein
Right brachial vein
Right basilic vein
Right median cubital vein
Right radial vein
Right median vein
Right cephalic vein
Right ulnar vein
Right femoral vein
Right popliteal vein
Right anterior tibial vein
Right posterior tibial vein

Left external jugular vein
Left internal jugular vein
Left brachiocephalic vein
Superior vena cava
Inferior vena cava
Left common iliac vein
Left internal iliac vein
Left external iliac vein
Left long saphenous vein
Left long saphenous vein
Left short saphenous vein

pushed outwards. The wall of the vein will become stretched and cause varicose veins.

Venous return

- The blood pressure in veins is low and constant.

- Pressure in the venules is approximately 16 mm Hg/kPa.

- Pressure in the right ventricle of the heart is 0 mm Hg/kPa.

- The pressure difference is normally sufficient to cause venous blood to return to the heart.

- When standing, the pressure pushing blood up and back to the heart is just enough to overcome the force of gravity. Two other mechanisms are used to help with venous return: (a) the skeletal muscle pump and (b) the respiratory pump.

Skeletal muscle pump

Contraction of leg muscles, due to movement, compresses the veins in the leg. The valve below the contracted muscle will close and the valves above (closest to the heart) will open upon pressure. The compression caused by the contracted muscle pushes blood up through the valve. This action is also called 'milking'. When muscles relax, the pressure falls causing the valve that is closer to the heart to close. The valve below will open as the blood pressure in the foot pushes the blood up.

The respiratory pump

When you breathe in (inspiration), the chest cavity (thorax) expands and creates a vacuum (negative pressure), drawing blood into the large veins. In addition, as the thorax expands, the diaphragm descends causing the pressure in the abdominal cavity to rise. This squeezes the veins and helps to push the venous blood up towards the heart.

Skeletal muscle pump

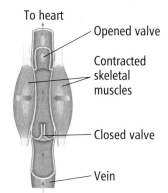

To heart

Opened valve

Contracted skeletal muscles

Closed valve

Vein

The graph below shows blood pressure changes as blood flows through the systemic circulation and the pulmonary circulation.

Blood pressure

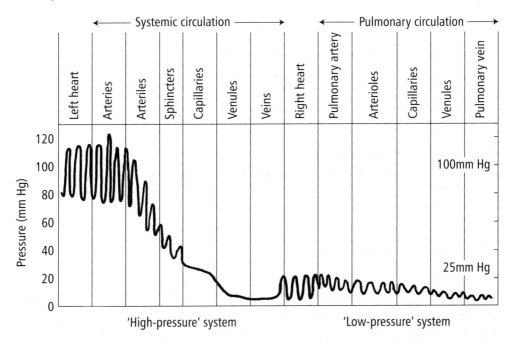

7 Functions and composition of blood

The human circulatory system contains blood, a fluid connective tissue that transports dissolved substances around the body. It is a sticky (viscous) red liquid that has many cellular components suspended in fluid. Temperature of blood is usually about 38 °C. The normal total blood volume depends on body weight. An adult male weighing 65 kg will have approximately 5 litres of blood; females will have slightly less. Blood is slightly alkaline and constitutes approximately 8% of a person's total body weight. The total volume of blood will contain 45% blood cells and 55% plasma.

The percentage of the total blood volume occupied by red blood cells is called the haematocrit.

A sample of blood collected in a test tube and spun in a centrifuge will separate into three layers:

- Plasma (55%).

- Red blood cells (45%).

- White blood cells and platelets called the buffy coat (less than 1%).

This laboratory investigation is used to show the measurement of haematocrit. This shows the percentage of red blood cells a person has in their blood.

Blood components

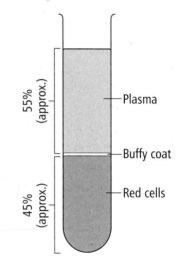

There will be a decrease in the number of blood cells if a person suffers from major blood loss following an accident, surgery, disruption in the cardiovascular system or problems associated with blood clotting (haemostasis).

Functions of blood

Transportation

- Blood carries oxygen and nutrients to cells throughout the body.

- It moves carbon monoxide from cells to the lungs.

- It carries heat and waste products away from cells.

- It transports hormones from endocrine glands, and enzymes to other body cells to activate homeostatic action.

- Blood will provide transport for harmful agents such as parasites and microorganisms so that they can travel around the body. Healthcare workers need to exercise great care to avoid unnecessary exposure to blood bourne microorganisms such as the human immunodeficiency virus (HIV) and hepatitis viruses that are transmitted via direct contact.

Regulation

- Blood maintains body temperature using the heat-absorbing and coolant properties of water in blood plasma. Heat distribution is assisted by the blood flow through the skin structure.

- Blood maintains pH levels (the symbol for hydrogen ion concentration that indicates the acidity/alkaline levels), fluid and electrolyte balance necessary for homeostasis.

Protection

- Blood protects the body from excessive blood loss by clot production (coagulation).

- It protects against infection and disease using platelets, white cells and proteins. Individuals who are obese have a greater volume of adipose tissue. Adipose tissue has a poor blood supply and therefore the transportation of nutrients and platelets, white cells and protein to injured areas will be affected causing delayed healing times.

Composition of blood

The circulating blood is composed of plasma and blood cells.

Plasma

- Straw-coloured, slightly alkaline fluid.
- 90% water.
- 8% plasma protein.
- 2% hormones, enzymes, nutrients, inorganic ions and waste.

Plasma proteins

There are many different plasma proteins in the blood. The proteins that are the most abundant are:

- Albumins: which accounts for 54% of plasma protein. Albumins help to maintain osmotic colloid pressure which is an important factor in the mechanism of the exchange of fluids across capillary walls. Albumin is responsible for making the plasma sticky in order to produce the viscosity of blood.

- Globulins: which account for 38% of plasma protein. These proteins include antibodies or immunoglobulins that produce a defence immune response against bacteria and viruses by creating antibodies.

- Fibrogens: which account for about 7% of plasma protein. Fibrogen is the key protein required in blood coagulation.

The composition of plasma

Blood plasma 55%		Formed elements 45%	
Proteins 8%	Albumins 54% Globulins 38% Fibrogen 7% Others 1%	Red blood cells 99%	
Water 90%		Platelets 1%	
Other substances	Electrolytes Hormones Nutrients Gases Vitamins Waste products	White blood cells 1%	Neutrophils 70% Lymphocytes 25% Monocytes 3% Eosinphils 2% Basophils 0.5%

Blood cells

The formation of blood cells takes place in red bone marrow and this process is called hemopoiesis (hē′-mō-poy-Ē-sis).

There are three types of blood cells: red blood cells (erythrocytes), white blood cells (leucocytes) and platelets.

Erythrocytes/red blood cells (RBC)

Red blood cells consist of a selective permeable membrane called cytosol and most of the volume of the cell is filled with a protein called haemoglobin. Haemoglobin carries oxygen and a red pigment that is responsible for the colour of blood. The red blood cell is unique in the human body as it is does not contain a nucleus.

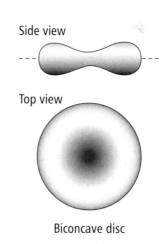

Side view

Top view

Biconcave disc

Red blood cells are produced in the red marrow of the long bones. As they have no nucleus they cannot divide and their replacement involves the production of millions of cells every minute.

Production of red blood cells

Production is stimulated by the hormone erythropoietin (eh-rith-rō-Poy-eh-tin).

If the body has low oxygen levels (hypoxia) the kidneys release erythropoietin into the circulation. Erythropoietin stimulates the red bone marrow to increase production of red blood cells. The increased number of red blood cells increases the oxygen-carrying potential of blood. When homeostasis is restored the kidneys reduce the amount of erythropoietin released.

Red blood cells are biconcave disks that provide a large surface area for gaseous exchange. Each cell is approximately eight-thousandths of a millimetre (8 μm) in diameter. Each red blood cell contains molecules of haemoglobin. The red-pigmented haemoglobin molecule is responsible for the transportation of respiratory gases and the acid/alkaline balance of blood (blood pH). There are approximately 200–300 million haemoglobin molecules in a mature red blood cell. Red blood cells live for approximately 120 days before being destroyed. Any remaining haemoglobin is recycled.

Haemoglobin molecule with iron ions

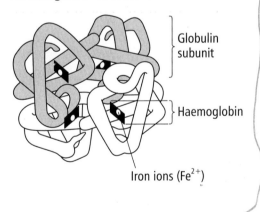

Globulin subunit

Haemoglobin

Iron ions (Fe^{2+})

Haemoglobin levels are recorded by grams of protein per 1000 cm^3 blood. In women the average reading is 12–16 g; in men it is slightly higher at 14–18 g due to their higher level of testosterone which stimulates production of more red cells.

If the number of red cells in the circulation falls or there is a reduced haemoglobin level, thus reducing the amount of oxygen delivered to the body cells, anaemia or circulatory problems will occur. To maintain the red blood cell count the body must receive appropriate quantities of vitamin B12, iron, protein and folic acid.

Leucocytes/white blood cells (WBCs)

White blood cells come in different forms and are produced in red bone marrow. All white blood cells are also called leucocytes (loo-kō-sı̄ ts) help to maintain the body's defences. Bacteria or viral infections or inflammation of tissue caused by trauma will cause the levels of the appropriate leucocytes to increase rapidly.

The two main types of white blood cells are:

- **Granular leucocytes** (three types): **Neutrophils, basophils and eosinophils**

  - Neutrophils: their main function is to engulf and destroy foreign bodies.

Neutrophils

  - Basophils: contain histamine and heparin and are involved in inflammatory or allergic reactions.

Basophils

  - Eosinophils: combat inflammation caused by allergic reactions and are effective against some parasitic worms.

Eosinophils

- **Agranular leucocytes** (two types):

  - Lymphocytes: these cells start immediate immune responses. There are three types of lymphocyte: *B cells* which secrete antibodies; *T cells* which attack viruses, cancer cells or transplanted tissue; and *natural killer cells* that attack infectious microbes.

Lymphocytes and monocytes

Lymphocytes

  - Monocytes: these enter the body tissue and become known as macrophages. Macrophages secrete substances that help to regulate the activity of the immune system and also digest

Monocytes

    foreign material and damaged body tissue in a process called phagocytosis.

The process of phagocytosis

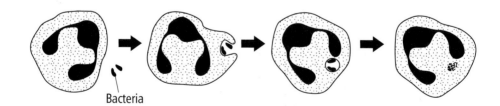
Bacteria

The white blood cells circulate around the body to locate any foreign pathogens in the system. The number of white cells varies, and there is a dramatic increase if a pathogen is located. White blood cells are chemically attracted to any site where inflammation has occurred (chemotaxis). A white cell has a life span of approximately 4–5 days.

Monocytes recognise bacteria and surround it. Once ingested the bacteria are digested by enzymes.

The monocyte will die up to 12 hours after phagocytosis has occurred.

Platelets

Platelets (thrombocytes) are formed in the bone marrow and are cellular fragments of a large megakaryocyte (megā-car′-e-o-sīt) cell. Thrombocytes are vital in haemostasis as they participate in the formation of clots.

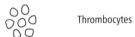

Thrombocytes

The thrombocytes and the walls of the damaged vessel release an enzyme called thrombokinase.

Thrombokinase starts the production of a mesh of protein strands formed by the thrombocytes trapping red blood cells and making a barrier. The barrier will help to prevent excessive blood loss from damaged vessels and also stop dangerous pathogens entering through damaged skin. The thrombocyte clot will be strengthened by additional coagulation methods that involve other proteins including fibrogen. The coagulation is a complex process as it relies on enzymes to trigger different stages of clot development.

Formation of a blood clot

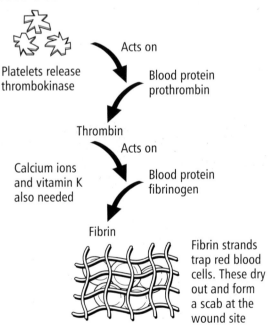

Platelets release thrombokinase

Acts on

Blood protein prothrombin

Thrombin

Acts on

Calcium ions and vitamin K also needed

Blood protein fibrinogen

Fibrin

Fibrin strands trap red blood cells. These dry out and form a scab at the wound site

Haemostasis

The process of haemostasis controls bleeding from any small blood vessels. Damage to the endothelial layer of blood vessels triggers messages that are sent in the blood to activate the four stages of haemostasis:

1   Seconds after an injury occurs the blood vessel will constrict (vasoconstriction) to limit the blood flow and blood loss so that the injury can be plugged by platelets (thrombocytes).

2   Thrombocytes will adhere to the damaged blood vessel (aggregation) and this triggers the complex process of clotting.

3   Clotting (coagulation) involves 13 different proteins that are activated to form a network of proteinous fibres containing thrombocytes and red blood cells. This forms a clot or thrombus.

4   As healing occurs, protein in the thrombus contracts bringing the edges of the wound closer together. When healing is complete an enzyme will break down the clot and the debris will be removed by phagocytic cells. This final stage of haemostasis is called fibrinolysis.

8 Blood groups and rhesus factors

There are approximately 35 identified blood groups with over 100 antigens. The principal blood-group systems are the ABO and rhesus factor.

Blood groups depend on the presence of proteins called isoantigens. Two antigens, A and B, are the basis of ABO blood groups.

Antigens are found on the surface membrane of red blood cells. If the red cell does not have a particular antigen an antibody will be produced if that missing antigen is placed in the blood, for example during a blood transfusion. The isoantibodies found in plasma will attack the antigen and cause the 'foreign' blood cells to clump together (agglutination) and block the blood vessels.

Antigens and antibodies

Blood type	Type A	Type B	Type AB	Type O
Red blood cell	A antigen	B antigen	Both A and B antigens	Neither A nor B antigens
Plasma	Anti B antibody	Anti A antibody	Neither antibody	Both anti A and anti B antibodies

Blood group A will have red cells with the antigen A on the surface membrane. The plasma will contain anti B antibodies. Anti B antibodies will attack antigen B.

Blood group B will have red cells with the antigen B on the surface membrane. The plasma will contain anti A. Anti A antibodies will attack antigen A.

Blood group O has neither antigen and may be given to any group.

Blood group AB has no antibodies and can be given to any group depending on the rhesus antigen.

The rhesus antigen D is present on the red cells of approximately 85% of the population. If this antigen is present the blood will be rhesus positive (rh+ve); if not it will be rhesus negative (rh−ve). Antibodies will occur if rh+ve blood is exposed to rh–ve blood. Antibodies are formed after the first exposure and reactions will occur if there is a second exposure following blood transfusion or a pregnancy with a rh+ve fetus and a rh–ve mother.

Anti D formation during pregnancy

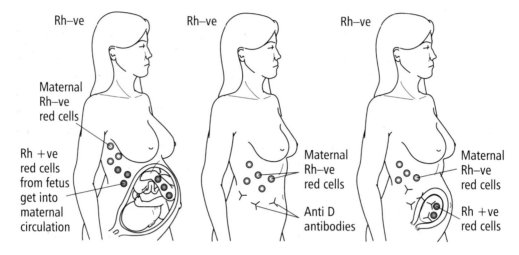

- First pregnancy exposes rh–ve mother to rh+ve cells .

- Mother produces anti D antibodies against rh+ve.

- Subsequent pregnancy will allow anti D antibodies to cross the placental barrier and attack rh+ve cells in the fetus.

To prevent this occurring all mothers are screened for rhesus status. An injection of anti D immunoglobulin following the birth of the baby will prevent the production of anti D antibodies.

9 Diseases and disorders of the circulatory system and blood

Anaemia

Anaemia is when the body's haemoglobin levels are low due to decreased red cell mass. Haemoglobin is a protein that is present in red blood cells and it is responsible for carrying oxygen around the body. A reduced oxygen-carrying capacity of the blood may lead to heart failure, peripheral vascular disease, cerebral anoxia (reduced oxygen to the brain causing dementia) and/or hypothermia (low body temperature). Symptoms of anaemia include fatigue, palpitations, headache, loss of appetite and breathlessness. There are many causes of anaemia and treatment depends on the underlying cause.

Iron deficiency anaemia

This is a common form of anaemia and may be due to dietary deficiency, problems with absorption (malabsorption) or blood loss.

The commonest causes are blood loss due to heavy periods (menorrhagia) or bleeding from the gastrointestinal tract (caused, for example, by an ulcer or cancer).

Pernicious anaemia

This anaemia is often associated with conditions such as thyroid disease and cancer of the stomach, but there are also congenital and genetic links. It is quite a rare anaemia but more common in northern countries. It is caused by the malabsorption of vitamin B12 due to a lack of gastric intrinsic factor. B12 deficiency may also lead to the peripheral nerves, bowel and tongue being affected.

Haemolytic anaemia

Anaemia is caused by an abnormally high rate of destruction of erythrocytes. Haemolytic anaemia may be due to inherited defects (sickle cell anaemia, thalassaemia) or acquired (due to infections, or if a person has a genetic deficiency of an enzyme which makes them susceptible to anaemia if they ingest certain drugs or poisons).

Deep vein thrombosis (DVT)

This is a blood clot (thrombus) situated in a deep vein of a leg. The clot may break off and travel through the circulatory system. If the clot is large it may occlude the pulmonary veins and cause a pulmonary embolism. This may cause total occlusion of a major vessel and lead to a cardiac arrest – when the heart stops beating due to lack of oxygen.

Hypertension

Blood pressure that remains raised at systolic 140/90 mm Hg diastolic is called hypertension. This is a common disorder in industrialised societies and is a major cause of heart failure, strokes and kidney disease. Treatment includes drug therapy and a lifestyle that avoids smoking, excessive alcohol and salt intake, and a diet that is high in fat and low in fibre and nutrients. Physical exercise and stress-relief techniques may help to lower blood pressure.

White-coat hypertension

This relates to the situation where blood pressure becomes raised only while being examined in a clinical setting by healthcare personnel.

Varicose veins

Varicose veins are caused by a defect of the valves in the veins. Valve damage may be congenital or acquired as a result of the valves being subject to high pressure following conditions caused by, for example, standing for long periods, obesity and pregnancy. Blood is allowed to flow back against the valve causing a pool of blood to form. The blood may then leak into the surrounding tissue causing swelling. Varicose veins occur in the veins close to the surface of the skin of the legs, oesophagus (oesophageal varices) and around the anus (haemorrhoids).

Further reading

Acheson, Sir D. (1998) *Report of the Independent Inquiry into Inequalities in Health*. Department of Health. The Stationery Office Ltd, London.

Department of Health (1998) *Our Healthier Nation: A Contract for Health*. The Stationery Office Ltd, London.

Ford, S. and Richards A. (1995) *GNVQ Human Physiology and Health in the Caring Context*. Nelson Thornes, Cheltenham.

Taylor, C., Lillis, C. and LeMone, P. (1997) *Fundamentals of Nursing: The Art and Science of Nursing Care*, 3rd edn. Nelson Thornes, Cheltenham.

References

Department of Health (1999) *Saving Lives: Our Healthier Nation*. The Stationery Office Ltd, London.

(Information is also available on the government website www.doh.gov.uk./hpss/index.)

Chapter 4

The nervous and endocrine systems

National unit specification
These are the topics you will be studying for this unit.

1   The nervous system

2   Structure of the nervous system

3   Disorders of the nervous system

4   The endocrine system

5   Disorders of the endocrine system

Diagrams to practise
Neuron
Synapse
Simple reflex arc
Positions in the body of the endocrine glands

Your learning outcomes may include the presentation of experiments in the form of written reports or data compiled and presented in graph form.

You will need to demonstrate knowledge of the basic anatomy and functions of the nervous and endocrine systems and their relevance and application to healthcare.

Homeostasis

The nervous and endocrine systems work closely together to regulate body processes and maintain homeostasis. The systems have different structures but they are not entirely separate entities. The hypothalamus controls the endocrine system; it is part of the autonomic nervous centre situated in the brain.

The nervous system controls homeostasis through nerve impulses and the endocrine system uses hormones.

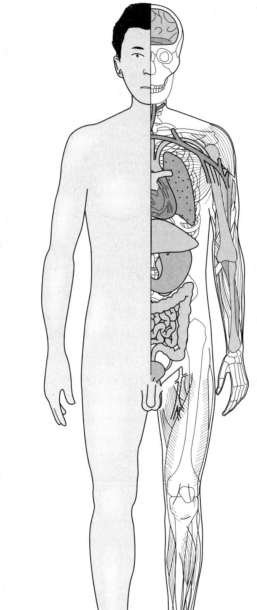

The nervous and endocrine systems

The nervous system	The endocrine system
Controls contraction of hair follicles	Stimulates hair growth and the sebaceous glands
Stimulates secretion from sweat glands	Stimulates bone growth
Pain receptors warn of damage in bone tissue	Stimulates the growth and development of the nervous system
Stimulates contraction of skeletal muscle	Increases blood flow to skeletal muscle during exercise
Controls muscle tone	Hormones control the level of calcium, glucagons and insulin necessary to maintain metabolism in muscle fibre
Regulates secretion of hormones from the adrenal glands and pancreas	Influences the growth and development of the nervous system
Governs heart rate and blood pressure	Elevates blood pressure during exercise or stress
Stimulates immune system	Reduces the inflammation and immune responses
Aids respiratory rate	Dilates the airways during exercise or stress
Helps to regulate digestion	Reduces the activity of the digestive system
Influences the amount of urine produced	Regulates blood volume by controlling the amount of fluid excreted as urine
Responsible for bladder control	Helps to control the amount of sodium and potassium in the blood
Influences sexual behaviour	Regulates the development, growth and secretions of the ovaries and testes

Both systems are involved with:

- Stimulus: to detect any changes in the external or internal environment.

- Receptors: organs that detect a specific message or stimulus.

- Effectors: organs, muscles or glands that produce a response following stimulus detection.

1 **The nervous system**

The nervous system has three main functions:

- Sensory functions: it receives information.

- Integrative functions: it processes information.

- Motor functions: the activation of relevant organs.

The nervous system consists of two types of cells:

- Neurons: for information processing.

- Neuroglia: to support and protect the neurons.

A nerve is made up of hundreds of neurons.

Neurons

- 10 billion neurons are present in the human body.

- Neurons are unable to divide or replicate.

- Neurons form connections with each other and body organs.

- The neuron is a specialised cell that is able to receive, process and transmit stimuli by means of an electrical charge.

Structure of a neuron

All neurons have a similar basic structure.

Nerve fibres that are covered with a myelin sheath are called medullated or white nerve fibres. Nerve fibres without a myelin sheath are called grey nerve fibres.

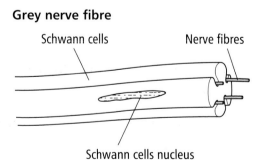

Grey nerve fibre

Schwann cells

Nerve fibres

Schwann cells nucleus

White nerve fibre

Nucleus
A

Cell body (centron)

Cytoplasm containing Nissl's granules, mitochondria, etc B

Cell membrane

Dendron C

Dendrites D

Axoplasm E

Thin membrane surrounding axoplasm F

Myelin sheath G

Schwann cell H

Neurilemma I

Node of Ranvier J

Axon

Direction in which impulse is transmitted

Terminal dendrites

Synaptic end bulb of axon

A	=	Purple
B	=	Light blue
C	=	Orange
D	=	Dark blue
E	=	Pink
F	=	Brown
G	=	Yellow
H	=	Red
I	=	Green
J	=	Maroon

* Diagram to practise

Cell body (or centron)

- Contains a nucleus that is surrounded by cytoplasm.

- Cell bodies vary in size and shape.

Two types of processes extend out from the cell body: dendrites and axon.

Dendrites

- The receiving or input portion of the neuron.

- Usually short and tapered, forming many branches called the dendritic tree.

Axon

- Conducts impulses towards another neuron or body cell.

- It is a long, thin, cylindrical projection that often joins the cell body at a small elevation called the axon billock.

- Some neurons have axons that are up to one metre long.

- Electrical charges that pass along the axon are called the action potential.

- The electrical charges are produced by ions, the most important ones being sodium (Na^+) and potassium (K^+).

- At rest, the surface membrane of the neuron has more positive charges on the outside and more negative charges in the cytoplasm (this is called polarisation).

- An impulse is activated when the balance of the charges is reversed (this is called depolarisation).

- Depolarisation continues down the neuron until repolarisation occurs.

Transmission of the nerve impulses

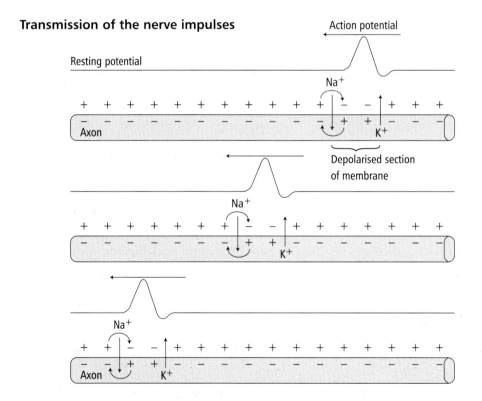

Synapse

The sites where neurons communicate are called synapses. There are two types of synapses: electrical and chemical.

Synapse-chemical

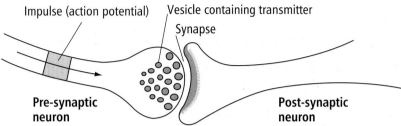

The axon bulb of the neuron that has action potential has a store of transmitter substance.

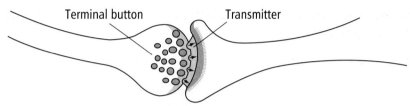

When the axon potential reaches the bulb the vesicle bursts open to release transmitter substance.

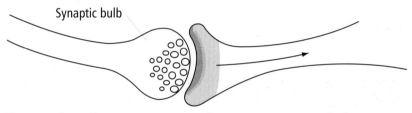

The transmitter substance moves across the synapse to receptors in the next neuron to create axon potential.

- The synapse is the area between one neuron's axon and another neuron's cell body or dendrite.

- The axon terminates in tiny branches with an end bulb. Within the end bulb are sacs (vesicles) that contain a chemical substance called a transmitter.

- Transmitter substances may differ but the main chemicals are acetylcholine and noradrenaline.

- The axon bulb is positioned close to a receptor in another neuron. The microscopic gap between the two is called the synaptic space.

- When action potential travels down the axon and reaches the axon bulb it causes the vesicle to burst open and release the transmitter substance.

- The transmitter substance moves across the synaptic space to the receptors in the other neuron. Concentrations of calcium and sodium alter to allow the transmitter to cross the synaptic space.

- The transmitter substance binds to the receptors and causes a change in the electrical potential of the axon due to increase in sodium ions.

- The action potential will keep occurring in the axon until the effect of the transmitter substance is stopped by the release of an enzyme into the synaptic space.

- Where synapses occur between nerves and muscles, a contraction of muscle will occur following action potential.

- There are many drugs that affect the neurotransmitters. Alcohol blocks the release of transmitters across the synapses, especially in the brain, and reactions and responses are slowed down.

The reaction and responses to specific stimulus may be a muscle reflex. This is a rapid and involuntary response and is created by the reflex arc. It is the reflex arc that causes a person to withdraw their hand automatically after touching a very hot object.

Reflexes

Simple reflex actions are present at birth and will result in the same responses occurring, often as protective behaviour. If an object approaches your face you will blink – a simple reflex action. The pathways that control a simple reflex are called simple reflex arcs.

If the response to stimuli is governed by learned behaviour, involvement of the nervous pathways and cerebrum of the brain is necessary to act on conscious thought. Learned behaviour is complex as it involves a variety of response stimuli.

Simple reflex arc

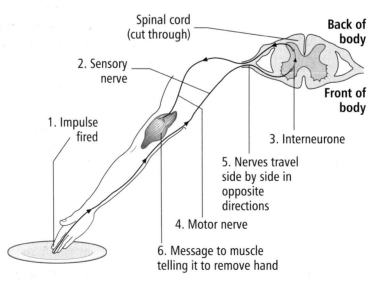

* Diagram to practise

2 Structure of the nervous system

The nervous system is responsible for communication throughout the body. Information is transmitted by the nerves of the peripheral nervous system, in the form of electrical pulses, to the brain. The information is then collated for storage or responded to by the central nervous system.

The nervous system

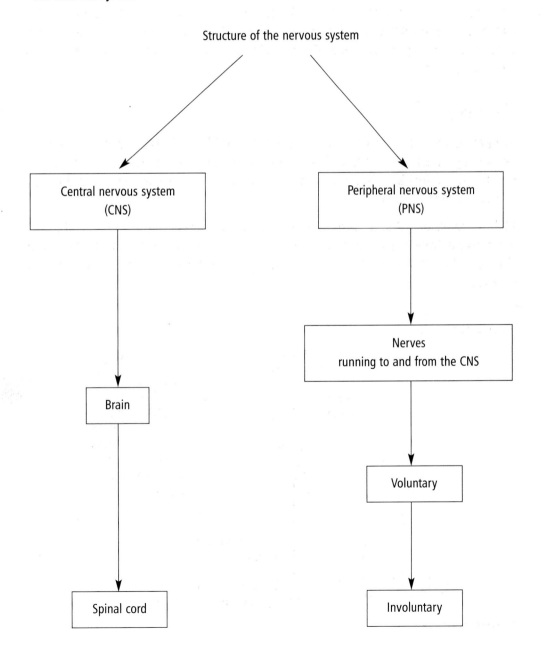

Central nervous system

The central nervous system consists of the brain and the spinal cord.

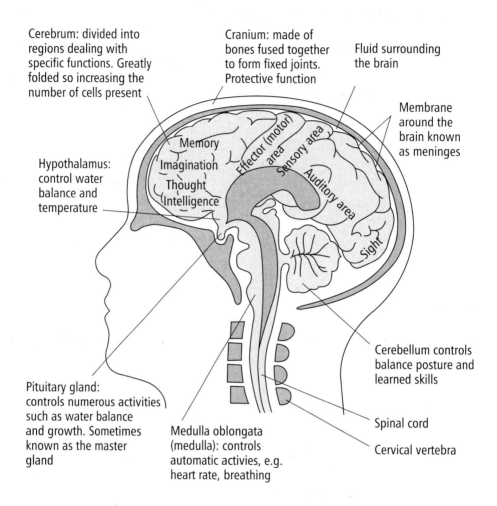

Cerebrum: divided into regions dealing with specific functions. Greatly folded so increasing the number of cells present

Cranium: made of bones fused together to form fixed joints. Protective function

Fluid surrounding the brain

Membrane around the brain known as meninges

Hypothalamus: control water balance and temperature

Memory
Imagination
Thought
Intelligence

Effector (motor) area

Sensory area

Auditory area

Sight

Cerebellum controls balance posture and learned skills

Pituitary gland: controls numerous activities such as water balance and growth. Sometimes known as the master gland

Medulla oblongata (medulla): controls automatic activies, e.g. heart rate, breathing

Spinal cord

Cervical vertebra

Meninges

The brain and spinal cord are surrounded by a membrane, called the meninges. There are three layers of the meninges:

- The dura mater: fibrous tissue that forms two layers within the skull. There is a potential space between the layers called the subdural space.

- The arachnoid mater: a delicate serous membrane. There is a potential space between the arachnoid and the pia called the subarachnoid space.

- The pia mater: a fine vascular layer attached to the brain. It protrudes into the ventricles and forms the choroid plexus that secretes cerebrospinal fluid.

Cross section showing the meninges

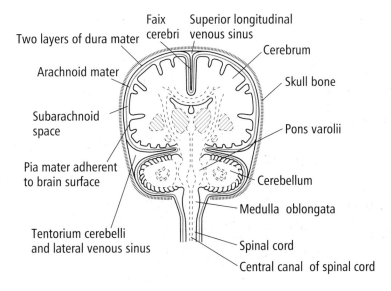

The ventricles

Within the brain are four cavities called ventricules that contain cerebrospinal fluid.

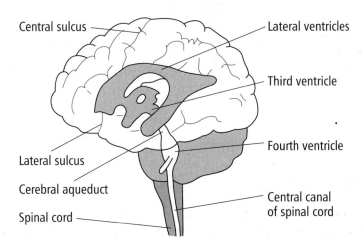

Cerebrospinal fluid (CSF)

Cerebrospinal fluid is a clear fluid similar to plasma and it contains water, mineral salts, glucose, proteins, urea and creatinine. It is formed from blood by the action of the choroid plexus which is situated in the third, fourth and lateral ventricles. The total volume of CSF in the system is usually about 200 ml at any one time. The fluid flows around the brain and spinal cord in the subarachnoid space before being reabsorbed into the blood via the arachnoid granulations and veins of the epidural space.

Functions of cerebrospinal fluid include:

- Supporting and protecting the brain and spinal cord.

- Maintaining a constant uniform pressure around the brain and spinal cord.

- Acting as a shock absorber.

- Keeping the brain and spinal cord moist and allowing transfer of substances between the fluid and nerve cells.

- Forming a medium for exchange between blood and brain, keeping the brain's biochemical environment constant even if changes occur in the blood.

Cerebrospinal fluid

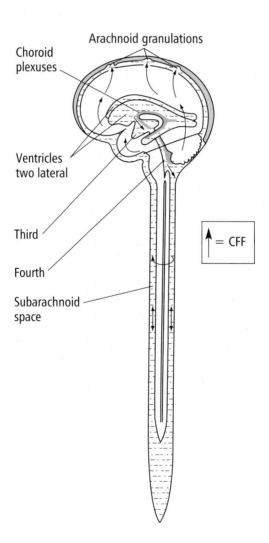

The brain

The brain is the nervous tissue that lies within the cranial cavity (skull). The following structures form the brain:

The cerebrum

- This is the largest part of the brain and it is divided into lobes.

- The grey matter of the cerebrum is on the outer layers and is known as the cortex. It is divided into two distinct parts either side of a deep cleft to form the right and left cerebral hemispheres.

- The cortex has many ridges/convolutions known as gyri, which are separated by sulci (a sulcus is a groove or depression; sulci – plural). The convolutions allow for a greatly increased surface area of grey matter.

- Deep within the brain the two hemispheres are joined by white matter (nerve fibres).

- The three main functions of the cerebral cortex are:
  - Mental activities involved in memory and intelligence.
  - Sensory perception of touch, sight, hearing, taste and smell.
  - The initiation and control of movement of voluntary muscle.

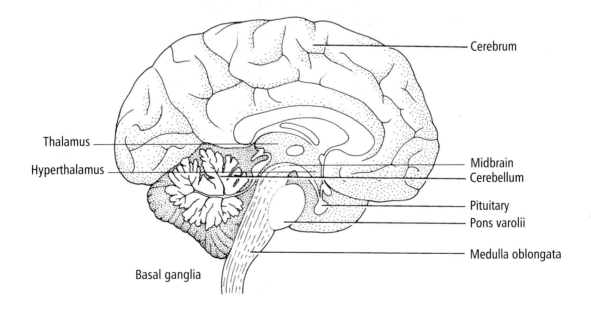

Anterior view of basal ganglia, thalamus and hypothalamus

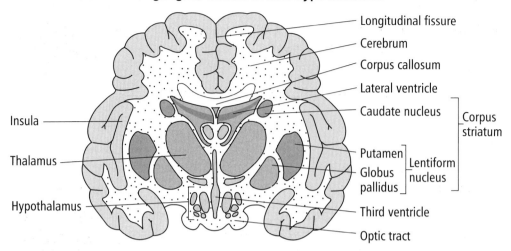

Basal ganglia

This is an area of grey matter that influences skeletal muscle that lies within the white matter of each cerebral lobe. It controls subconscious movement and muscle tone. The largest paired area of basal ganglia is the corpus striatum.

The thalamus

- A mass of nerve cells that collect information from all sensory nerves located in the peripheral areas of the body.

- It provides an awareness of touch, pain and temperature but is unable to distinguish finer sensations.

The hypothalamus

- It controls and integrates the activities of the pituitary gland and the autonomic nervous system.

- It regulates emotional and behaviour patterns.

- It controls body temperature.

- It regulates eating behaviour.

- It helps to maintain sleep patterns.

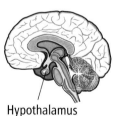

Hypothalamus

The mid brain

- This consists of nerve cells and fibres that connect with lower parts of the brain and the spinal cord.

- It relays motor impulses from the cortex to the pons.

- It relays sensory impulses from the spinal cord to the thalamus.

Mid brain

114

The pons varolii

- This forms a bridge between the two hemispheres of the cerebrum to relay messages from one side to the other.

- It works with the medulla to help control breathing.

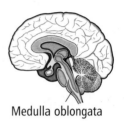

Pons

The medulla oblongata

- It relays impulses between other parts of the brain and the spinal cord.

- Vital centres are present in the deeper structure which regulate the cardiac cycle, blood vessel diameter and the respiratory centre.

- It coordinates centres involved in stimulating the reflex centres for vomiting, coughing, sneezing and hiccupping.

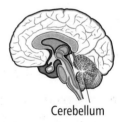

Medulla oblongata

The cerebellum

- It coordinates activities to maintain the balance and equilibrium of the body.

- It also coordinates complex skilled movement below the level of consciousness.

Cerebellum

The peripheral nervous system

The peripheral nervous system is all nerves outside of the brain and spinal cord. The peripheral nerves allow messages to be transmitted to and from the central nervous system and consists of:

- 12 pairs of cranial nerves.

- 31 pairs of spinal nerves.

- The autonomic part of the nervous system.

Cranial nerves

The cranial nerves connect directly with the brain and do not pass through the spinal cord. The cranial nerves are named according to their function or by a conventional numbering system.

Cranial nerve	Function	Tissues involved
(I) Olfactory	Sensory	Nose
(II) Optic	Sensory	Retina of eye
(III) Oculomotor	Motor	Muscles that move the eyes and upper lip
(IV) Trochlear	Motor	Superior oblique muscle of the eye
(V) Trigeminal	Sensory	Orbits of the eye, nasal cavity and forehead
Maxillary	Sensory	Skin of the face, upper lips, gums, teeth and palate
Mandibular	Mixed – sensory	Skin of the jaw, lower gums, teeth and lip
	– motor	Muscles used in chewing (mastication) and floor of the mouth
(VI) Abducens	Motor	Lateral muscles of eyes
(VII) Facial	Mixed – sensory	Tongue
	– motor	Facial muscles used in expression; salivary and tear glands
(VIII) Vestibulocochlear	Sensory	Ear
(IX) Glossopharyngeal	Mixed – sensory	Pharynx, tongue, carotid arteries and aortic arch
	– motor	Pharynx – swallowing, salivary glands
(X) Vagus	Mixed – sensory	Pharynx, larynx, oesophagus, thorax and abdomen
	– motor	Pharynx, larynx, oesophagus, thorax and abdomen
(XI) Accessory	Motor	Pharynx, larynx and soft palate (swallowing) Muscles of the neck
(XII) Hypoglossal	Motor	Tongue

Cranial nerves

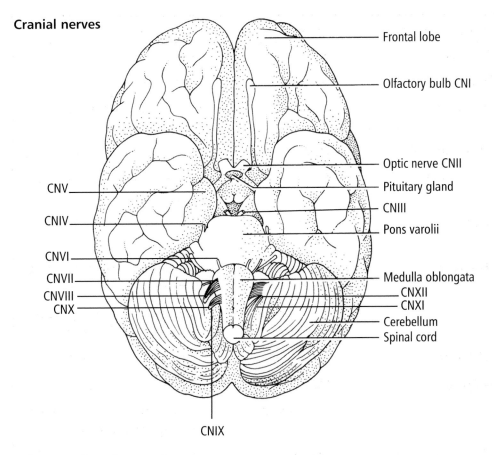

The spinal cord lies within the vertebral canal of the vertebral column. It is the nervous tissue link between the brain and all the organs of the body.

Functions of the spinal column

- It transmits motor activity from the brain to target tissues within the body.

- It carries sensory activity from around the body to the brain.

- The outer section consists of white matter that has fibres which go up and down the spinal cord.

- At each vertebral joint in the spine there is a space for nerve roots to enter or exit, forming the spinal chord roots.

- The fibres of the white matter are highly organised and form columns called dorsal, lateral or ventral columns depending upon location.

- Within the columns the neurons passing information to a specific area of the brain are arranged into distinct tracts.

- Collectively the tracts are called spinothalmic tracts.

- The inner section of the cord contains grey matter that consists of neuronal cell bodies, axons and glial cells.

Spinal column

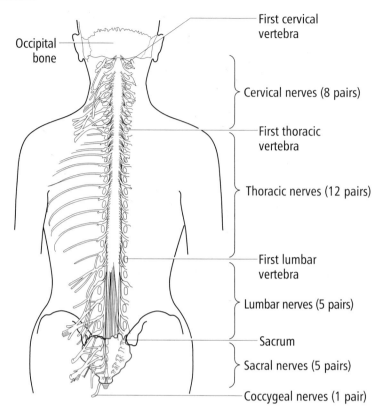

Occipital bone

First cervical vertebra

Cervical nerves (8 pairs)

First thoracic vertebra

Thoracic nerves (12 pairs)

First lumbar vertebra

Lumbar nerves (5 pairs)

Sacrum

Sacral nerves (5 pairs)

Coccygeal nerves (1 pair)

- The grey matter processes and/or relays incoming information from sensory neurons and outgoing motor activity, and it plays an integrative role in reflex responses.

- The spinal canal lies at the centre of the cord and extends into the medulla of the brain. Here it communicates with the fourth ventricle of the brain.

- The spinal canal is filled with cerebrospinal fluid (CSF) that circulates up and down the canal.

- The fluid provides a protective environment for the spinal column, providing hydraulic support and shock absorbance.

Spinal nerves

The nerve roots leave the cord at specific intervals. At each vertebral joint there is a pair of posterior and anterior nerve roots. The nerve roots fuse together after leaving the cord, in the spaces between the vertebrae, forming the spinal nerves.

Structure of the spinal cord

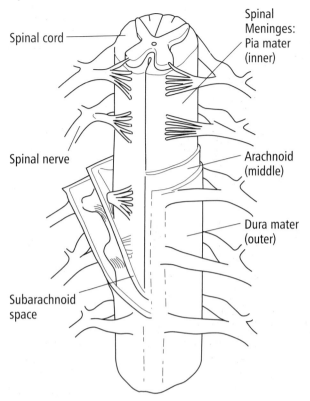

Spinal nerve

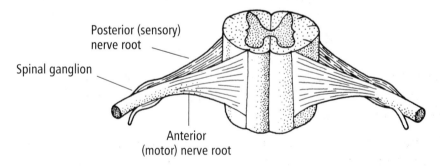

There are 31 pairs of spinal nerves, each consisting of sensory and motor neurons:

- Cervical vertebrae: eight pairs of spinal nerves.

- Thoracic vertebrae: twelve pairs of spinal nerves.

- Lumbar vertebrae: five pairs of spinal nerves.

- Sacral vertebrae: five pairs of spinal nerves.

- Coccygeal vertebrae: one pair of spinal nerves.

The paired spinal nerves provide pathways to specific areas of the body. The areas or segments that are linked to a particular spinal nerve are called dermatones.

Dermatones

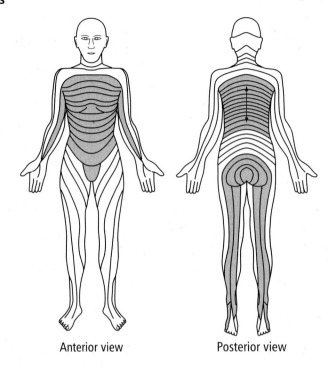

Anterior view   Posterior view

The autonomic nervous system

The autonomic nervous system controls the functions of the internal organs and tissues of the body. The system functions at an unconscious and involuntary level. The autonomic nerves will activate or inhibit activity. An individual autonomic nerve will have the ability to either increase or decrease the activity of tissue cells (it cannot do both). This function is vital to maintain homeostatic control of the internal environment. The autonomic nervous system is divided into the sympathetic and parasympathetic pathways that produce opposite effects on tissue cells.

Sympathetic pathways

- Sympathetic nerves leave the spinal canal between the sixth cervical and second lumbar vertebrae.

- The nerves run into the sympathetic ganglia that lies alongside the spinal column.

- Changes in the sympathetic nerve activity occur during periods of stress caused by factors such as exercise or the 'flight or fight' response. The excitatory response will have an overall effect on responses to maintain cellular homeostasis.

- Changes that may occur include:
  - Increase in cardiac output – increased heart rate.
  - Vasodilation of muscles to increase blood flow.

The sympathetic pathways

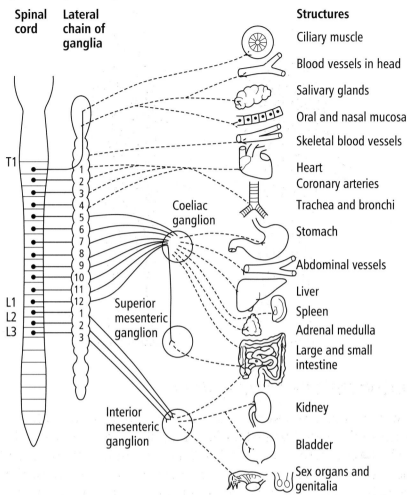

- Pupils dilate to enhance peripheral vision.
- Sweat secretion is stimulated to remove excess heat produced by the raised metabolic rate.
- Glycogen stores are released from the liver and muscle to provide glucose as fuel.
- Reflexes are enhanced to promote rapid movement.
- The bronchules dilate to facilitate lung ventilation.
- Activity of the gut is inhibited.

Parasympathetic pathway

- The parasympathetic pathway consists of the cranial nerves and nerves in the region of the sacrum.

- The vagus nerve contains parasympathetic fibres that reach the main body organs, excluding the urinary, genital and lower digestive system.

- To inhibit action of an organ, the parasympathetic nerves synapse with efferent nerves in the intramural ganglia that are situated alongside the organs. Neurons in the target areas receive the message from the efferent nerves.

The parasympathetic pathways

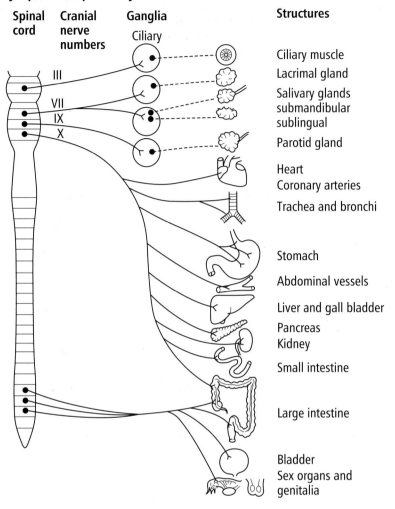

Spinal cord	Cranial nerve numbers	Ganglia	Structures

The effects of the parasympathetic and sympathetic nervous system

Organ or system	Sympathetic	Parasympathetic
Eye	Dilates pupil	Constricts pupil
Salivary glands	Concentrated secretion stimulated	Watery secretion stimulated
Sweat glands	Increased production	No known effect
Cardiovascular system	Vasodilation of muscle	
Blood vessels	Vasoconstriction of vessels in the skin and digestive viscera	No known effect
Blood pressure	Increases	Decreases
Heart rate	Increases	Decreases

Organ or system	Sympathetic	Parasympathetic
Adrenal gland	Secretes adrenaline and noradrenaline via the medulla	No known effect
Respiratory system		
Diameter of airways	Increases	Decreases
Respiratory rate	Increases	Decreases
Digestive system		
Sphincter muscles	Contract	Relax
Activity	Decreases	Increases
Secretory glands	Inhibited	Stimulated
Urinary system		
Kidneys	Decreases the production of urine	No known effect
Bladder	Relaxes muscle of the bladder	Contracts muscle of the bladder
	Contracts internal sphincter	Relaxes internal sphincter
Sex organs	Ejaculation of semen	Vasodilation

Sensory input

The nervous system allows sensory input from organs connected with smell, taste, vision, hearing and balance. To maintain homeostatic balance in our environment we also need to collect input on temperature, textures, pain, position of our body and condition of internal organs.

For the body to react to any sensation, consciously or unconsciously, a series of events must occur:

- A stimulus must be present to activate relevant sensory neurons.

- A sensory receptor is then able to convert the stimulus to a nerve impulse.

- The nerve impulse must then be conducted along the nerve pathway to the brain.

- The brain receives and interprets the impulse, turning it into a perceived sensation.

Sensory pathways

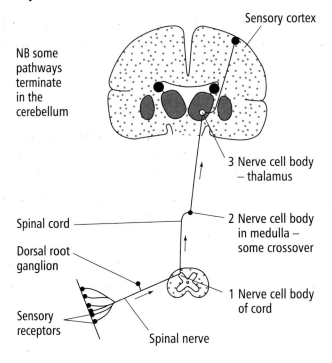

NB some pathways terminate in the cerebellum

Sensory cortex

3 Nerve cell body – thalamus

Spinal cord

2 Nerve cell body in medulla – some crossover

Dorsal root ganglion

1 Nerve cell body of cord

Sensory receptors

Spinal nerve

Sensory receptors are varied and carry different stimulus. A sensory receptor will carry information about one type of sensation only. Light, heat, pressure, mechanical energy or chemical energy are stimuli that activate receptors.

Senses are grouped into two categories: general and special senses.

General senses

General senses are divided into two groups.

Somatic senses:

- Touch, pressure and movement/vibration.
- Hot and cold.
- Pain.
- Joint and muscle position.
- Movement of the head and limbs.

Pain receptors are located in nearly all body tissue. Referred pain is that felt when the sensation of pain is sent to the skin from an organ nearby (irritation of the diaphragm causes referred pain in the shoulder area).

Visceral senses:

- These provide information about internal organs and body fluids.

Special senses

Receptors for special senses of smell, sight, hearing, equilibrium and taste are more complex in structure than general senses and are found in specific receptor organs – nose, eyes, ears and tongue.

Location of sensory receptors

- Exteroceptors (eks'-tēr-ō-SEP-tors): located in the skin or near the surface of the body to provide information about the external environment – vision, sound, smell, taste, touch, temperature, pressure and pain.

- Interoceptors (in'-ter-ō-SEP-tors): located in blood vessels and organs. These provide information about the internal environment – pain, fatigue, nausea, pressure, hunger and thirst.

- Proprioceptors (pr-ō'-prē-ō-SEP-tors): located in muscles, joints and the ear. These provide information about body movement and position.

3 Disorders of the nervous system

Acute meningitis

Meningitis is an infection of the pia mater and arachnoid. It carries a high mortality rate and diagnosis is made by examining a sample of cerebrospinal fluid. Early high doses of appropriate antibiotics will reduce the mortality rate. The organisms causing acute meningitis vary depending on a person's age. Children over four years of age are more likely to suffer from meningococcus infection, while adults are more susceptible to pneumococcus.

Clinical features

- Rapid development of fever with reduced alertness.

- Increasingly severe headache.

- Sensitivity to light (photophobia).

- Purpuric rash: this rash spreads rapidly and does not fade when pressure is applied.

- Meningism: signs of meningeal irritation that include pain and resistance when the chin is flexed down towards the chest.

Meningitis is more common in areas of poverty, overcrowding and malnutrition. It may follow a head injury, sinusitis, ear infection, a surgical procedure that involves CSF (shunts or lumbar punctures), and conditions where the body's immune system is suppressed (AIDs, cancer, sickle-cell disease). Vaccines against meningitis are now available but the vaccine does not protect against all organisms that cause pyrogenic meningitis ('pyro' means heat or fever).

Cerebrovascular incident (CVI)

Cerebrovascular incidents occur following:

- any interruption of the blood supply to the brain; or

- any injury to the nerve cells and/or nerve pathways within the brain; or

- any increase of pressure in the cranium

causing the loss or reduction in function of the part of the brain that has been affected. A cerebrovascular incident (also known as a stroke) may occur at any age but it is more common in later years. It is potentially fatal and is the third leading cause of death in the western world.

Factors that increase the risk of CVI are:

- High blood pressure.

- High blood cholesterol levels.

- Smoking.

- Heart disease.

- Obesity.

- Excessive alcohol intake.

Clinical features

- Usually a sudden onset causing loss of consciousness due to haemorrhage from a cerebral artery.

- The pressure of leaking blood on the motor pathways interrupts nerve impulses.

- Damage in the motor cortex of one side of the cerebral hemisphere will cause weakness or paralysis in the opposite side of the body. Weakness of one side of the body is called hemiparesis and paralysis is called hemiplegia.

- Pressure of leaking blood on the sensory pathways interrupts impulses returning to the brain.

- Damage to the sensory cortex will cause loss of feeling in one side of the body.

- Pressure within the cranium rises due to the bleeding and compresses the medulla oblongata. This will inhibit the swallowing and cough reflexes.

- Raised pressure within the cranium will compress the nerve centres and inhibit activity, causing changes in blood pressure, poor temperature control and respiratory distress.

- Damage to the cerebellum will affect coordination and balance. This will cause the person to have an unsteady gait which is called ataxia.

- Damage to the left cerebral hemisphere will affect speech (this is called dysphasia).

- Death will occur if the damage to the brain is severe.

Approximately 40 % of people will make a full recovery following a CVI. The remainder will display evidence of varying levels of neurological defects. Intense nursing care, physiotherapy and speech therapy will help people to recover some of the lost functions following a CVI and prevent complications such as contractures of joints, muscle wasting, constipation and depression.

Epilepsy

Epilepsy is indicated when there is intermittent abnormal electrical activity in the brain. This activity manifests itself as a seizure. The cause is not always found, but it may be due to physical or metabolic problems, infection, or a disease or syndrome.

Headaches

Headaches are a common complaint and the pain is caused by the stimulation of nerve ends in the scalp, sinuses, arteries or the periosteum of the skull. The brain itself has no pain sensors. The causes of headaches vary from tension or non-specific to the potentially fatal pain caused by raised intracranial pressure created by infection or haemorrhage.

Multiple sclerosis

Multiple sclerosis (MS) is a chronic disorder that is characterised by the formation of small plaques and changes in the myelin sheath throughout the central nervous system. This occurs in recurrent episodes. Relapses may last a few months and remissions may last for years. MS is more common in temperate climates with distinct regional variations of prevalence. Clinical features may include weakness of the legs, deterioration of central vision, vertigo, double vision, pain and incontinence. There is no cure at present and the sufferer will need to adjust to live with varying levels of disability.

Transient ischaemic attacks

Transient ischaemic attacks (TIA) are local disturbances of the central nervous system caused by small blood clots (emboli) or blocking (occlusion) of a blood vessel. The symptoms last for up to 24 hours. TIAs may be a warning sign of future strokes or heart attack.

Clinical features

- An abrupt onset of neurological features (i.e. symptoms that affect the nervous system) that fade over minutes or hours to give a full recovery within 24 hours.

- Symptoms depend on where the clot or occlusion has occurred and may include:
    - Weakness of one side of the body.
    - Dysphasia.
    - Vertigo.
    - Deafness.

- Vomiting.
- Ataxia.

Treatment for transient ischaemic attacks will be aimed at control of the risk of further clots or occlusion.

4 The endocrine system

There are two types of glands in the body: endocrine and exocrine. Exocrine glands secrete directly into ducts and include sweat, sebaceous mucus and digestive glands. These glands are not part of the endocrine system.

The internal environment of the body is controlled partly by the autonomic nervous system and partly by the endocrine system.

The two systems provide a means of communication between the different parts of the body and coordinate tissue and organ function to maintain homeostasis.

The endocrine system consists of ductless glands that secrete hormones into the bloodstream via the interstitial tissue. Each gland produces a chemical substance called a hormone which is able to affect target cells in a specific organ and influence their activity, growth and nutrition. Hormones usually stimulate activity of an organ.

The endocrine system consists of the following glands.

- Pineal body.
- Pituitary gland.
- Thyroid gland.
- Four parathyroid glands.
- Two adrenal glands.

Organs that contain cells that that secrete hormones include the hypothalmus, thymus, pancreas, ovaries, testes, kidneys, stomach, liver, small intestines, skin, heart, placenta and adipose tissue. They differ from endocrine glands in that they have ducts which carry secretions directly in to the relevant body organs.

The position of the endocrine glands

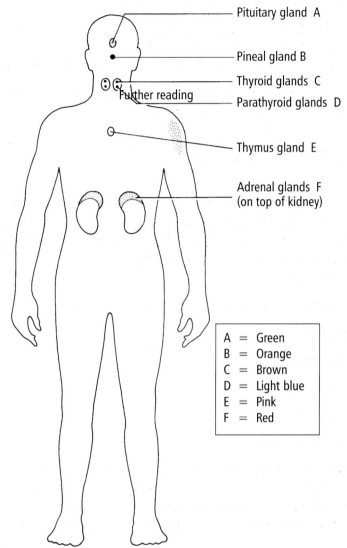

Pituitary gland A

Pineal gland B

Thyroid glands C

Further reading

Parathyroid glands D

Thymus gland E

Adrenal glands F
(on top of kidney)

A = Green
B = Orange
C = Brown
D = Light blue
E = Pink
F = Red

* Diagram to practise

Functions of hormones

Hormones help to regulate:

- Volume and composition of extracellular fluid.
- Metabolic rate and energy balance.
- Biorhythm: the body's biological clock.
- Contraction of smooth muscle.
- Contraction of cardiac muscle.

- Secretion from glands.

- The immune system activities.

- Control the growth and development of the body.

- Control the functions of the reproductive systems.

Responses that are coordinated by hormones tend to be slower than responses coordinated by the nervous system.

Hormone secretion is regulated by:

- Signals from the nervous system.

- Chemical changes in the blood.

- Other hormones.

How hormones work

Target cells

Hormones are secreted into the interstitial fluid and then into the bloodstream or interstitial tissue. The hormones will only become active when they reach specific cells which are able to chemically bind with the hormone. The receptor cells are called target cells and are composed of protein molecules.

Hormones are divided into two groups:

- Lipid soluble: steroid and thyroid hormones.

- Water soluble: adrenaline, histamines, melatonin, human growth hormone and insulin.

The way in which a hormone works will depend upon whether it is lipid or water soluble. Lipid soluble hormones enter the cells before binding to the receptors and the reaction to the hormone is slow. Water soluble hormones act by relaying messages from target cells that activate the release of several enzymes which produce physiological responses.

Hormones may be released into the circulatory system or into localised areas.

Hormones and their receptor cells

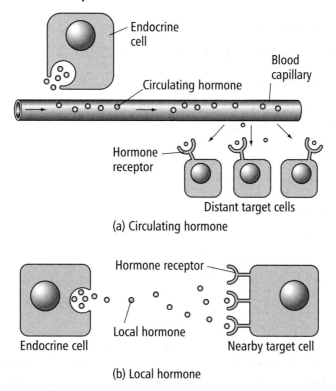

(a) Circulating hormone

(b) Local hormone

Negative feedback

Most hormone release is regulated by a system called negative feedback. If the level of a particular hormone falls, it turns on the mechanism to release more of that hormone into the blood. If the level of hormone rises it will turn off the mechanism.

When hormones are no longer needed they are made inactive by the liver, kidneys and lungs and then excreted in the urine.

Control of hormone secretions

Factors that regulate hormone secretion include:
- Messages from the nervous system.

- The change in chemical balance in the blood.

- Messages from other hormones.

The release of hormones is regulated to prevent over- or under-production.

Pituitary gland

The pituitary gland is situated in a depression of the sphenoid bone at the base of the brain. It is roughly oval in shape and divided into the anterior and posterior lobes. The gland is attached to the brain by a stalk called the infundibulum. Nerve fibres allow the hypothalamus and pituitary to communicate with each other. The hypothalamus is the major link between the endocrine and nervous system and plays a vital role in homeostasis and growth and development. The cells in the hypothalamus synthesize hormones and the pituitary gland secretes hormones.

Position of the pituitary gland

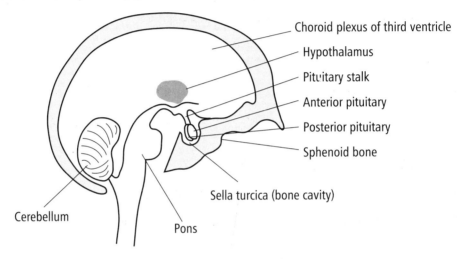

The anterior and posterior lobes of the pituitary gland are responsible for secreting and storing several different hormones.

Anterior pituitary hormones

Human growth hormone (HGH)

- Secretion is regulated by the hypothalamus.

- It stimulates liver, bone and other tissue to release growth factors for metabolism and general body growth.

- It affects the growth of long bones by promoting the growth of the epiphyseal cartilage.

Thyrotrophic hormone (TSH)

- It controls the growth and activity of the thyroid gland.

- The amount of TSH in the bloodstream is influenced by thyroxine levels (thyroxine is produced by the thyroid gland).

Follicle stimulating hormone (FSH) and luteinising hormone (LH)

These are also called sex hormones.
In men:

- FSH stimulates the production of sperm.

- LH stimulates the secretion of testosterone.

In women:

- FSH stimulates the development of the ovary follicle and secretion of oestrogen by the ovaries.

- LH stimulates the secretion of oestrogen and progesterone and triggers the discharge of the mature ovum (ovulation).

Prolactin (PRL)

- Responsible for growth and development of breasts during pregnancy.

- Promotes production and flow of milk from the mammary glands.

Adrenocorticotropic hormone (ACTH)

- Stimulates the adrenal gland to produce its hormones.

- The production of ACTH is important during periods of stress.

Melanocyte-stimulating hormone (MSH)

This is responsible for the production of melanocytes which affect the skin pigmentation (colour).

Posterior pituitary hormones

The posterior pituitary gland is composed of secretory cells and nerve fibres that are triggered by the hypothalamus. The pituitary gland stores hormones until it is triggered to secrete them.

The two hormones stored in the posterior pituitary gland are as follows.

Oxytocin

- Secreted before and during labour and when a baby is suckling.

- Promotes contraction of the uterus and stimulates lactation.

- May be partly responsible for producing the feeling of pleasure during and after sexual intercourse.

Antidiuretic hormone (ADH) or vasopressin

- Promotes the kidneys to increase the amount of water returned to the blood, reducing the amount of urine produced.

- Dehydration and overhydration influence secretion of ADH.

- Other factors that affect ADH production are stress, pain, drugs, smoking and alcohol.

The thyroid gland

The thyroid gland lies at the front (anterior) of the neck and consists of two lobes that lie either side of the trachea. The lobes are joined by a narrow band of thyroid tissue called an isthmus.

The thyroid gland is extremely vascular and each lobe is approximately 5 cm long and 3 cm wide. Each lobe contains microscopic thyroid follicles of follicular cells that produce two hormones, thyroxine (thīROK-sēn) and triiodothyronine (trī-ī-ōdō-THī-rō-nēn). Smaller parafollicular cells are situated in the thyroid and produce the hormone calcitonin (kal'-si-TŌnin).

Action of thyroxine and triiodothyronine

Iodine is present in blood and this is taken up by the gland to stimulate the production of thyroid hormones. Many body cells have receptors for thyroid hormones.

The effects of thyroid hormones are widespread throughout the body.

- Thyroid hormones are responsible for normal mental and physical development.

- They are responsible for maintaining healthy skin and hair.

- They influence the excitability of nerve fibres.

- They control how oxygen is used throughout the body and this regulates the basal metabolic rate and normal body temperature.

- They stimulates protein synthesis and help to reduce blood cholesterol levels.

- They stimulate the absorption of carbohydrates in the small intestines.

The hypothalamus stimulates the thyroid to release hormones during pregnancy, when cold and when there is low blood glucose to assist in homeostasis.

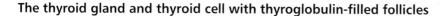

The thyroid gland and thyroid cell with thyroglobulin-filled follicles

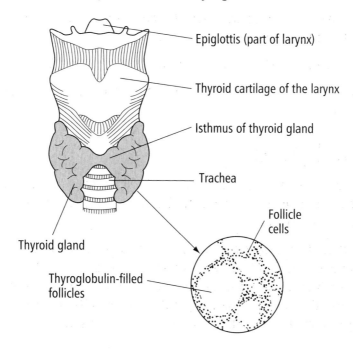

Epiglottis (part of larynx)

Thyroid cartilage of the larynx

Isthmus of thyroid gland

Trachea

Follicle cells

Thyroid gland

Thyroglobulin-filled follicles

Calcitonin

The secretion of calcitonin is controlled by a negative feedback system. Its function is to reduce the blood level of calcium by inhibiting the action of osteoclasts and the reabsorption of calcium from bones.

The parathyroid glands

The four parathyroid glands are located on the posterior surface of the thyroid gland. There are two parathyroid glands embedded in each thyroid lobe. The parathyroid glands are small oval-shaped structures and they secrete the hormone parathormone. The cells forming the glands are named principal cells and they are arranged in columns with channels containing blood between the columns.

Action of parathormone

- It keeps the blood concentration of calcium within normal limits by stimulating the kidney to reabsorb calcium. By activating vitamin D, it also increases the amount of calcium absorbed from food through the intestinal cells.

- It keeps the blood concentration of magnesium and phosphate ions within normal limits by stimulating the kidney to excrete excess phosphate and magnesium.

Parathyroid glands (viewed from behind)

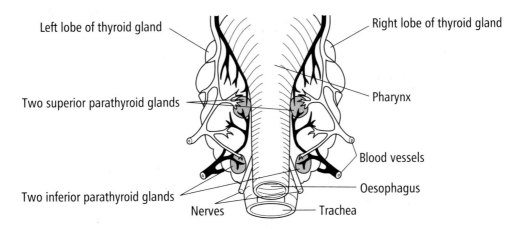

- Left lobe of thyroid gland
- Right lobe of thyroid gland
- Two superior parathyroid glands
- Pharynx
- Blood vessels
- Oesophagus
- Two inferior parathyroid glands
- Nerves
- Trachea

- It promotes the formation of the hormone calcitriol in the kidney. This hormone is an active form of vitamin D.

Parathormone is produced by negative feedback and its secretion is directly linked to blood calcium levels. The correct calcium levels are essential for nerve impulse transmission, blood clotting and effective muscle contraction.

The adrenal glands

The two adrenal glands are situated at the top of each kidney, surrounded by a capsule of tissue containing fat. Each adrenal gland is composed of two regions: the inner adrenal medulla and the outer adrenal cortex. The two sections of the adrenal gland differ anatomically and physiologically.

Adrenal medulla

This forms the smallest part of the adrenal gland and it is completely surrounded by the adrenal cortex. It consists of cells from the autonomic nervous system that specialise in secreting hormones. When stimulated by the sympathetic neurons the adrenal medulla produces two principal hormones: epinephrine and norepinephrine (also known as adrenaline and noradrenaline).

Actions of adrenaline and noradrenaline

Adrenalin and noradrenaline are produced as a response to danger, stress or excitement.

- They increase the blood supply to the heart by dilating the coronary arteries.
- They increase the amount of air reaching the lungs by dilating the bronchi.
- The amount of oxygen and nutrients to muscle is increased by dilating the blood vessels that supply skeletal muscle.

The adrenal glands

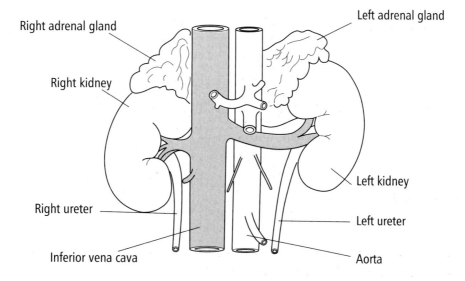

- Blood pressure is raised by constricting blood vessels to the skin.

- They stimulate muscle fibres of the iris to dilate the pupils of the eyes.

- Peristalsis action of the digestive system is slowed down.

- The amount of saliva and digestive juices produced is reduced.

- They inhibit passing of urine (micturition) and opening of bowels (defecation) by increasing the tone of the urethral and anal sphincters.

- They cause goose-bumps and an increase in the activity of the sweat glands.

Functions of the adrenal cortex

The adrenal cortex is divided into three areas that make and secrete different types of hormones: glucocorticoids, mineralocorticoids and androgens (sex hormones).

Glucocorticoid (gloo'-kō-KOR-ti-koyd)

Glucocorticoids affect glucose homeostasis. Hormones secreted are cortisol (hydrocortisone) and corticosterone, and functions include:

- Maintaining blood glucose levels.

- Stimulating the process of gluconeogenesis – the production of glucose from non-carbohydrate sources found in the liver.

- Increasing the rate of protein breakdown into amino acids for energy.

- Releasing fatty acids from adipose tissue.

- Providing additional glucose and causing a rise in blood pressure needed to maintain homeostasis during times of stress or abnormal internal/external environment.

- Inhibiting white blood cells that participate in the inflammatory process.

- Reducing the body's response to antigens.

- Decreasing the amount of calcium absorbed by the small intestines.

Mineralocorticoids (min'-er-al-ō-KOR-ti-koyds)

Mineralocorticoids aid homeostasis by helping to control water, sodium and potassium levels. The main hormones are aldosterone (al-DOS-ter-ōn) and angiotensin (an'-jē-ō-TEN-sin).

Aldosterone:

- Stimulates the reabsorption of sodium via the renal tubules.

- Increases the amount of potassium excreted.

- The sodium and potassium levels affect the amount of water reabsorbed.

Angiotensin stimulates the secretion of aldosterone when there is a fall in the level of blood sodium.

Androgens (sex hormones)

In males and females the adrenal cortex secretes androgens. The secretion of hormones is controlled by adrenocorticotropic hormone (ACTH) and functions of androgens include:

- Influencing the development of secondary sex characteristics in males and females – growth of axillary and pubic hair, pre-puberty growth spurt.

- Increasing the deposit of proteins in muscles.

- In females: conversion of oestrogen from other body tissue, this being the only source of oestrogen following the menopause.

- Contributing to sex drive (libido) in females.

- In males the sex hormone testosterone is produced by the testes. Testosterone regulates the production of sperm and stimulates the development of masculine characteristics.

- In females the ovaries produce oestrogen and progesterone. These hormones are responsible for the development of feminine characteristics and also help to regulate the menstrual cycle. The hormones are also active in maintaining pregnancy.

- In pregnancy the placenta has endocrine functions. Oestrogen is produced from the placenta in large amounts throughout pregnancy to promote changes in physiology to support fetal development. Human chorionic gonadotrophin (HCG) is produced in early pregnancy to help maintain oestrogen and progesterone levels.

Pineal body

The pineal gland (PIN-ē-al) is a small reddish structure situated deep within the brain.

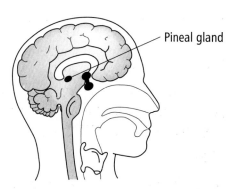

Pineal gland

Functions

The function of the pineal gland is not yet fully understood. Historically the pineal body was thought to be the spiritual centre of the brain. Hormones known to be produced by this gland are:

- Melatonin: the amount released is based on daily cycles (circadian rhythms) relating to the amount of light entering the eye – levels are high at night and low in the day. It helps to regulate sleep.

- Histamine.

- Dopamine.

The pineal gland calcifies during adulthood to reduce its effectiveness in old age.

Endocrine cells

Hormones produced by organs other than glands but that contain endocrine cells include:

Gastrointestinal tract

- Gastrin: promotes secretion of gastric juices.

- Glucose-dependent insulintropic peptide: stimulates the release of insulin.

- Secretin: stimulates secretion of pancreatic juices and bile.

- Cholecystokinin (ko'le-sis'to-kin'in): stimulates secretion of pancreatic juices and bile.

Placenta

- Human chorionic gonadotrophin: stimulates ovaries to produce oestrogen and progesterone.

Kidneys

- Erythropoietin (êh-rith'-rō-POY-eh-tin): increases the rate of production of red blood cells.

The pancreas

The pancreas is a soft pink gland situated in the upper abdomen and lies partly behind the stomach. It is a mixed gland that has endocrine and exocrine functions. The endocrine part of the pancreas is situated in clusters of endocrine cells called the islets of Langerhans.

The hormones produced by the islets of Langerhans are involved with the metabolism of glucose.

- Insulin: reduces blood glucose levels and affects fat and protein metabolism when the concentration of blood glucose is elevated.

- Glucagon: causes an elevation of blood sugar levels. The brain requires a constant supply of glucose and if levels fall, brain damage may occur.

- Somatostatin: moderates the release of insulin and glucagons, preventing excess secretion.

- Pancreatic polypeptide: helps to regulate the release of digestive enzymes from the pancreas.

Anterior view of pancreas

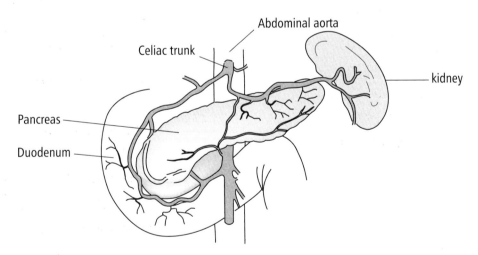

Islets of Langerhans

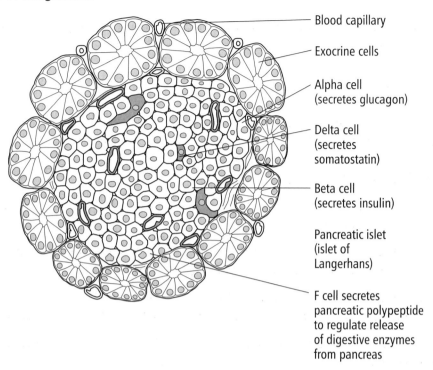

- Blood capillary
- Exocrine cells
- Alpha cell (secretes glucagon)
- Delta cell (secretes somatostatin)
- Beta cell (secretes insulin)
- Pancreatic islet (islet of Langerhans)
- F cell secretes pancreatic polypeptide to regulate release of digestive enzymes from pancreas

Endocrine function of Islet of Langerhans

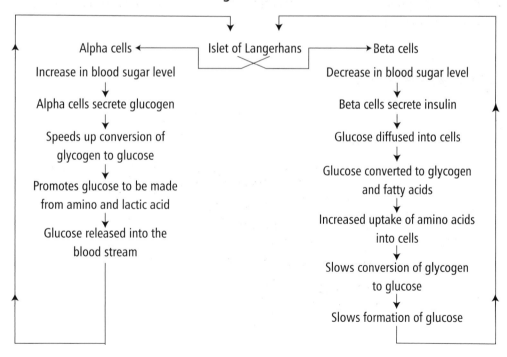

Alpha cells ← Islet of Langerhans → Beta cells

Alpha cells	Beta cells
Increase in blood sugar level	Decrease in blood sugar level
Alpha cells secrete glucogen	Beta cells secrete insulin
Speeds up conversion of glycogen to glucose	Glucose diffused into cells
Promotes glucose to be made from amino and lactic acid	Glucose converted to glycogen and fatty acids
Glucose released into the blood stream	Increased uptake of amino acids into cells
	Slows conversion of glycogen to glucose
	Slows formation of glucose

The thymus gland

The thymus gland is situated behind the sternum and consists of two lobes. The thymus produces hormones to stimulate the development of T lymphocyctes (white cells that destroy microbes and debris). The thymus gland becomes smaller during adulthood and is replaced by connective tissue in old age. The hormones released by the thymus are:

- Thymin.

- Thymosin.

- Thymopoietin.

These hormones all have similar actions but the mechanism for their control is not yet been fully identified.

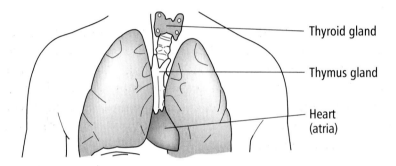

Thyroid gland

Thymus gland

Heart
(atria)

5 Disorders of the endocrine system

Disorders of hormone function are due to:

- The body's failure to control hormonal secretion.

- A lack of response of the target cells to the hormones.

Pancreas

Diabetes mellitus

Diabetes mellitus is the most common endocrine disease. There are two types of diabetes:

- Type 1 – insulin dependent: caused by the immune system destroying the insulin-producing cells which leads to a constant high blood sugar level and glucose being excreted in the urine. This condition is usually seen in children and requires daily injections of insulin (either genetically engineered or from animal sources) to maintain homeostasis. Poor control of blood sugar levels affects the blood vessels and nervous system, leading to severe damage of tissue and organs.

- Type 2 – non-insulin dependent: caused by an inadequate response to insulin supply by the body tissues (insulin resistance). Type 2 diabetes usually occurs in those over the age of 40 (though any age group is vulnerable), and there are approximately 1.4 million sufferers in the UK with a possible further 1 million being undiagnosed (Diabetes UK, 2003). It is often associated with obesity, high cholesterol levels and high blood pressure – this group of symptoms are called metabolic syndrome. Treatment includes weight reduction, dietary changes and alterations in lifestyle.

Pituitary gland disorders

Pituitary dwarfism

Undersecretion of the human growth hormone slows the rate of bone growth and the epiphyseal plates will close before the child's normal height is reached.

Pituitary gigantism

Oversecretion of human growth hormone during childhood will result in the long bones becoming abnormally long causing the child to grow very tall.

Thyroid

Graves disease (hyperthyroidism)

A high level of thyroid hormone will cause a person to become hyperactive. Clinical signs and symptoms include restlessness, agitation, inability to tolerate heat, rapid pulse, increased appetite and weight loss. Physical signs include swelling of the face and bulging eyes (due to swelling behind the eyes). The thyroid gland also swells and this is seen as a bulge in the neck area which is called a goitre (GOY-ter).

Myxoedema (mix'ō-DE-ma)

Low levels of thyroid hormones will cause slow heart rate, low body temperature, dry skin, muscle weakness, lack of energy and weight gain. Signs of myxoedema include swelling of the face, hands and feet, a goitre and a toad-like face. This condition affects more women than men.

Cretinism

Hyposecretion of thyroid hormones in young infants will result in cretinism. In pregnancy the level of thyroid hormones is controlled by the mother's thyroid and the fetus is affected by low levels of maternal thyroid hormones. Low levels of thyroid hormones in infancy may cause brain damage as the brain will fail to develop properly. The skeletal growth may also be affected causing dwarfism. If detected at an early stage, cretinism is preventable by the use of oral hormone therapy.

Further reading

Campion, K. (1997) Multiple sclerosis. *Professional Nurse* **13**(3),169–172.

Cree, L. and Rischmiller, S. (1991) *Science in Nursing*, 2nd edn. W. B. Saunders/Baillière Tindall, Sydney.

Gard, P. R. (1998) *Human Endocrinology*. Taylor and Francis, London.

Givens, P. and Reiss, M. (1996) *Human Biology and Health Studies*. Nelson and Sons, UK.

Greenfield, S. (2000) *The Private Life of the Brain*. Penguin, London.

Hinchliff, S. and Montague, S. (1998) *Physiology for Nursing Practice*. Baillière Tindall, London.

Tamir, E. (2002) *The Human Body Made Simple*, 2nd edn. Churchill Livingstone, Edinburgh.

Tortora, G. J. and Grabowski, S. R. (1993) *Principles of Anatomy and Physiology*, 7th edn. Harper Collins, New York.

Tortora, G. J. and Grabowski, S. R. (2001) *Introduction to the Human Body*, 5th edn. Wiley, New York.

Waugh, A. and Grant, A. (2001) *Ross and Wilson's Anatomy and Physiology in Health and Illness*, 9th edn. Churchill Livingstone, Edinburgh.

Internet sites

The Migraine Trust: www.migrainetrust.org

National Society for Epilepsy: www.epilepsynse.org.uk

Multiple Sclerosis Society: www.mssociety.org.uk

Brain and Spine Foundation: www.brainandspine.org.uk

British Brain and Spinal Foundation: www.bbsf.org.uk

Reference

Diabetes UK: www.diabetes.com

Chapter 5

The respiratory system

National unit specification
These are the topics you will be studying for this unit.

1   Organs of the respiratory system

2   The mechanism of breathing

3   The respiratory cycle

4   Diseases and disorders of the respiratory system

Diagrams to practise

The upper respiratory tract

Structure of an alveolus

Homeostasis

The function of the respiratory tract is to provide cells with oxygen and remove carbon dioxide. A healthy adult will breathe in approximately 14,000 litres of air a day. Oxygen is a vital substance necessary for homeostasis and if it is not provided cells will die within minutes.

Muscular system:
Allows for an increased rate and depth of breathing to supply muscles with additional oxygen during exertion.

Nervous system:
The nose provides an area for receptors for the sense of smell.
Inspiration of air provides vibrations necessary for speech from the vocal cords.

Endocrine system:
Promotes the production of the hormone angiotensin II that is used in the regulation of blood pressure.

Cardiovascular system:
Respiratory muscles help to pump venous blood into the heart.

Lymphatic and immune system:
Lining of the upper respiratory tract helps to trap debris and bacteria.
The tonsils contain lymph tissue.

Digestive system:
Voluntary contractions of the respiratory system assist defecation.

Urinary system:
The two systems work together to regulate the acid/alkaline balance of body fluids.

Reproductive system:
Increases oxygen supply during exertion.
Provides oxygen to fetus via internal respiration.

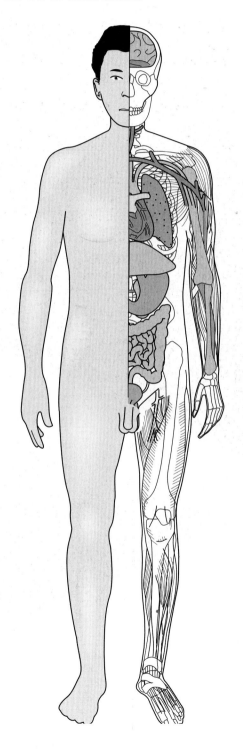

1 Organs of the respiratory system

The respiratory system and the cardiovascular system supply the body with oxygen and remove waste carbon dioxide. A failure in either system will result in rapid cell death. Respiration is achieved by ventilation, external respiration and internal respiration. It is important to identify the difference between ventilation and respiration.

- Ventilation (breathing): is the process of drawing air in and out of the lungs using muscles in the diaphragm and intercostal muscles (muscles between the ribs).

- Respiration: is the process that occurs inside cells. Oxygen is supplied to the cells for cellular respiration.

The respiratory system consists of organs that facilitate the exchange of gases between the atmosphere and the blood.

The respiratory system

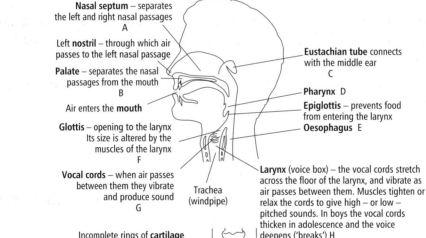

Nasal septum – separates the left and right nasal passages A

Left **nostril** – through which air passes to the left nasal passage

Palate – separates the nasal passages from the mouth B

Air enters the **mouth**

Glottis – opening to the larynx Its size is altered by the muscles of the larynx F

Vocal cords – when air passes between them they vibrate and produce sound G

Incomplete rings of **cartilage** support the trachea and bronchi

Thoracic cavity in which the lungs lie, protected by the ribs

The **trachea** divides into the left and right bronchi K

Right **lung**

Heart L

Diaphragm – a sheet of muscle that forms the base of the thoracic cavity

Eustachian tube connects with the middle ear C

Pharynx D

Epiglottis – prevents food from entering the larynx

Oesophagus E

Larynx (voice box) – the vocal cords stretch across the floor of the larynx, and vibrate as air passes between them. Muscles tighten or relax the cords to give high – or low – pitched sounds. In boys the vocal cords thicken in adolescence and the voice deepens ('breaks') H

Trachea (windpipe)

Ribs (in cross-section) I

Intercostal muscles (between ribs) J

The left **bronchus** passes to the left lung M

Pleural membranes N

Pleural fluid O

Abdominal cavity

Bronchiole / Alveoli } **Bronchial tree**

A = Green	E = Light pink	I = Yellow	M = Dark orange
B = Light orange	F = Red	J = Lilac	N = Dark pink
C = Brown	G = Dark blue	K = Grey	O = Light green
D = Light blue	H = Purple	L = Tan	

* Diagram to practise

The respiratory system consists of:

- The upper respiratory tract: nose, pharynx, larynx, trachea, bronchi and bronchioles.
- The alveoli.

Upper respiratory tract

The upper respiratory tract comprises of the airway from the nose to the alveoli.

Nose

- The nose is formed by two nasal bones and cartilage.
- The nasal cavity is divided by the septum. The nasal cavity is connected to the pharynx through two openings called the internal nares.
- The roof of the nose is formed by the ethmoid bone at the base of the skull, and the floor is formed by the hard and soft palates of the roof of the mouth.
- The nose is covered and lined by skin. Inside, the nose hairs help prevent foreign bodies entering the respiratory system.
- The cavity of the nose is lined with ciliated mucous membrane. This area is extremely vascular and atmospheric air is warmed as it passes over the epithelium.
- Mucous is produced that moistens air and entraps dust. The cilia moves the mucous along to the pharynx for swallowing or expectoration.

Pharynx

The pharynx is comprised of three sections:

- Naso-pharynx: lies behind the nose, the posterior wall is where the pharyngeal tonsil (adenoids) are situated.
- Oro-pharynx: lies below the level of the soft palate and this is where two pairs of tonsils are situated. The oro-pharynx is part of the respiratory and alimentary tract. It is not possible to swallow and breath at the same time because the oro-pharynx is blocked off from the nasal-pharynx by the raising of the soft palate when swallowing occurs.
- Laryngeal-pharynx: the larynx is composed of several irregular-shaped cartilages that are joined together by ligaments and membrane. Vocal cords stretch across the floor of the larynx and vibrate as air passes between them.
  - Thyroid cartilage: the thyroid cartilage is formed by two flat pieces of cartilage fused at the front to form the laryngeal prominence (the Adams apple).
  - The larynx increases in size during male puberty and this, together with variation in pitch caused by the vocal cords becoming thicker and stretched, causes the voice to become deeper.

Passage of air through the nose and pharynx

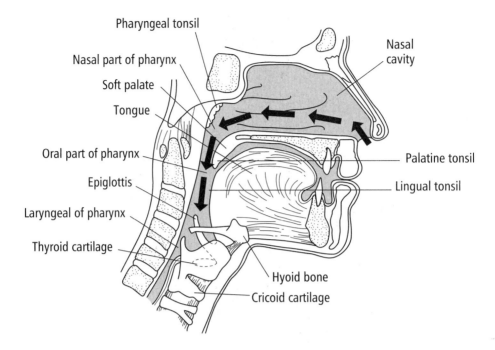

Trachea

- The trachea is lined with ciliated epithelia containing goblet cells that secrete mucous and sweep mucous and foreign particles upwards towards the larynx.

- The wall of the trachea is made of involuntary muscle and fibrous tissue strengthened by incomplete rings of hyaline cartilage. The tracheal cartilages are horseshoe-shaped to provide a rigid structure which is necessary to prevent the tube closing.

The vocal cords

- The oesophagus lies behind the trachea. There is no cartilage on the side of the trachea that is next to the oesophagus. This is to allow flexibility and permits food to pass through to the stomach. The lungs lie on either side of the trachea.

- The trachea begins below the larynx and travels down the front of the neck into the chest. There it divides into the left and right bronchi.

The trachea and associated structures

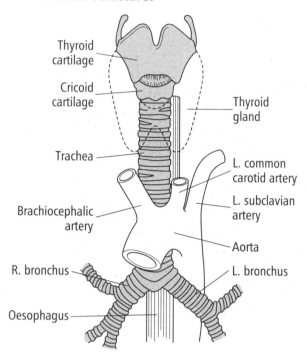

Bronchial tree

- The bronchi supply each of the two lungs. Each bronchi divides to form lobar bronchi to supply the two or three lobes of each lung. The lobar bronchi divide to form the segmental bronchi to supply self-contained broncho-pulmonary segments of each lung.

- As the bronchi become finer, the cartilage in their walls is replaced by muscle and elastin fibres (myoelastic).

- The tiny airways are called bronchioles and they continue to divide to form the terminal bronchioles, respiratory bronchioles and the alveolar ducts leading to the alveoli.

- The bronchi contain stretch receptors to prevent over-inflation of the lungs.

The bronchial tree

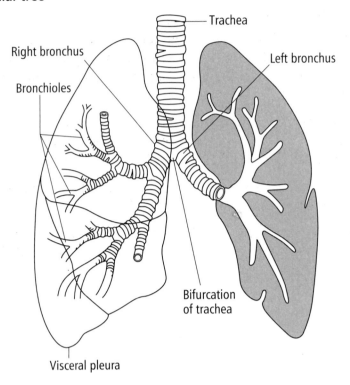

Lungs

The two lungs are cone-shaped and lie on each side of the thoracic cavity. The lungs are divided into lobes. The right lung has three lobes and the left lung has two lobes. Each lobe has its own blood supply and bronchi.

The lungs with associated structures

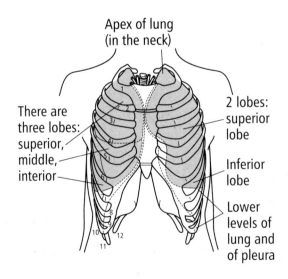

- The lungs are separated from each other on the medial surface by a space called the mediastinum.

- On the medial surface of each lung there is an area called the hilus where the pulmonary arteries and veins, lymph vessels, parasympathetic nerves, sympathetic nerves and the main bronchi enter the lung. This region is known as the root of the lung.

- The outside surface of the lungs is covered in a thin membrane called the visceral pleura. The pleural membranes also cover the inside of the thoracic cavity and the thoracic surface of the diaphragm, the parietal pleura.

- The pleural membranes are kept separated by a thin layer of serous fluid called pleural fluid.

- The pleural fluid prevents friction between the surfaces when breathing takes place. The pleural fluid occupies a potential space called the pleural cavity.

Medial view of the lungs

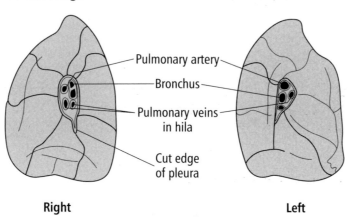

Pulmonary artery

Bronchus

Pulmonary veins in hila

Cut edge of pleura

Right   **Left**

The pulmonary blood supply

- The pulmonary artery divides into a right and left branch and carries deoxygenated blood to each lung.

- The exchange of gases between the air in the alveoli and the deoxygenated blood takes place in the capillary network surrounding the alveoli.

- The oxygenated blood leaves the lungs via the pulmonary veins to the left atrium of the heart.

Blood flow between the heart and lungs

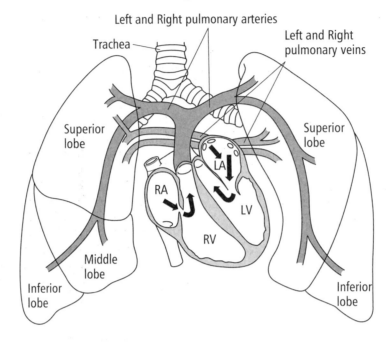

The exchange of gases between the alveoli and blood is influenced by the thickness of the walls of the alveoli and blood vessel and interstitial fluid between them. The movement of gases across this barrier is dependent upon pressure generated by individual gases within a gas mixture.

Air contains 21% oxygen, nitrogen, carbon dioxide and small amounts of other gases making up what is called total pressure of air. The individual gases give a partial pressure. Partial pressure depends on the proportion of gases present. Gases diffuse at different pressure gradients.

*Alveoli

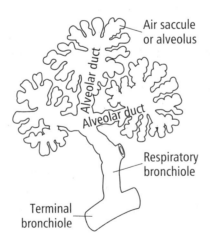

* Diagram to practise

Gas exchange in the lungs

Cluster of alveoli   **Section through alveolus showing gas exchange**

Air moves in and out

Bronchiole

Blood with a low oxygen concentration and a high carbon dioxide concentration

Blood with a high oxygen concentration and a low carbon dioxide concentration

Air moves in and out

Blood vessels from the pulmonary veins take blood enriched with oxygen from the alveoli to the heart

Gases dissolve in layer of moisture

Carbon dioxide diffuses out of blood
Oxygen diffuses into blood

Wall of capillary only one cell thick

Alveoli

Blood vessels from the pulmonary arteries bring blood with a low oxygen level from the heart to the alveoli

Wall of alveolus – only one cell thick

Key

➡ Transport of oxygen

⇨ Transport of carbon dioxide

Red = Blood with high oxygen concentration
Blue = Blood with low oxygen concentration

* Diagram to practise

Alveoli foundations

There are millions of microscopic alveoli that form air-filled cavities within the lungs creating a huge alveolar surface for the exchange of gases to take place.

- The walls of the alveoli are very thin and contain three cell types:
  - Phagocytic macrophages: which engulf and destroy microorganisms or debris.
  - Squamous epithelial cells: that form the wall of the alveoli.
  - Cuboidal epithelial cells: which secrete a fluid called a surfactant that moistens the membrane to reduce surface tension and prevents the alveoli collapsing.

- The alveoli are in close contact with capillaries, and oxygen passes from the air in the alveolar cavity into the blood. Carbon dioxide passes from the blood into the alveolar cavity. This process is called external respiration.

2 The mechanism of breathing

The mechanism of breathing is the process created when the lungs expand to take in air and then contract to expel air. The movement of air during breathing depends on the differences in pressure in the airways and atmospheric pressure. Air will flow from a high-pressure region to a low-pressure region.

- Inspiration: air is breathed in (inhalation) when the volume of the chest cavity increases. This causes the pressure in the chest cavity to fall below atmospheric pressure, so air is pushed into the lungs by the higher pressure.

- Expiration: air is breathed out (exhalation) when the volume of the chest cavity decreases. The pressure in the lungs becomes higher than the atmospheric pressure, so air is pushed out from the lungs.

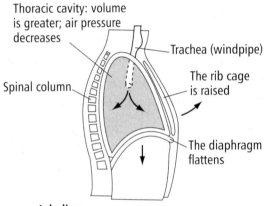
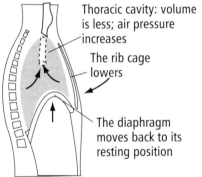

Thoracic cavity: volume is greater; air pressure decreases

Trachea (windpipe)

Spinal column

The rib cage is raised

The diaphragm flattens

Thoracic cavity: volume is less; air pressure increases

The rib cage lowers

The diaphragm moves back to its resting position

Inhaling
a) The intercostal muscles contract, lifting the ribs upwards and outwards
b) The diaphragm muscles contract and the diaphragm flattens
The movements increase the volume of the thoracic cavity. As a result the pressure of air inside the thoracic cavity decreases and becomes less than atmospheric pressure. Air, therefore, is drawn into the lungs

Exhaling
a) The intercostal muscles relax, letting the ribs drop downwards and inwards
b) The diaphragm muscles relax and the diaphragm returns to its resting position
The movements decrease the volume of the thoracic cavity, helped by the elastic recoil of the ribs and diaphragm returning to their resting positions. As a result the pressure of air inside the thoracic cavity increases and becomes greater than atmospheric pressure. Air, therefore, is forced out of the lungs into the trachea

The movement of air into the lungs relates to Boyle's law. This law states that at a constant temperature the pressure of a gas is inversely proportional to its volume.

Muscular activity is required to expand the thoracic cavity during inspiration. Muscular activity is a partially voluntary and partially involuntary action. The main muscles used during respiration are the intercostal muscles and the diaphragm.

Intercostal muscles

- There are 11 pairs of intercostal muscles that occupy the spaces between the 12 pairs of ribs.

- Contraction of the intercostal muscles pulls the ribs upwards and outwards which increases the volume of the chest cavity.

- The intercostal muscles are controlled by the medulla area of the brain stem.

Diaphragm

- The diaphragm forms the floor of the thoracic cavity and the roof of the abdominal activity.

- When relaxed, the diaphragm is a dome-shaped muscle.

- The muscle fibres radiate and are attached to the spinal column, the lower ribs and the sternum with a central tendon.

- As the diaphragm contracts during inspiration, the central tendon pulls the diaphragm down causing it to flatten. The volume of the chest cavity expands in a downwards direction.

- The diaphragm's nervous system is supplied by the phrenic nerves.

The intercostal muscles and the diaphragm contract at the same time, moving the pleural membranes to force the lungs to expand. This ensures that the thoracic cavity is enlarged in all directions and will create a drop in pressure, allowing air to enter the lungs.

Intercostal muscles

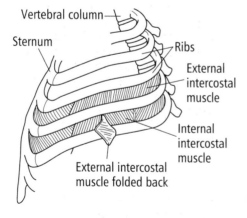

Vertebral column
Sternum
Ribs
External intercostal muscle
Internal intercostal muscle
External intercostal muscle folded back

Movement of the diaphragm

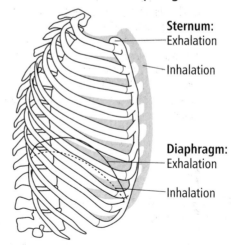

Sternum:
Exhalation
Inhalation

Diaphragm:
Exhalation
Inhalation

Muscles involved in the mechanism of breathing

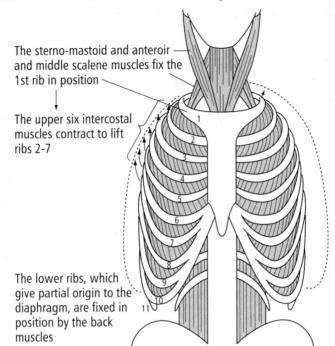

The sterno-mastoid and anteroir and middle scalene muscles fix the 1st rib in position

The upper six intercostal muscles contract to lift ribs 2-7

The lower ribs, which give partial origin to the diaphragm, are fixed in position by the back muscles

3 The respiratory cycle

During a period of quiet relaxed breathing, a healthy person will take approximately 14–18 breaths per minute. The volume of air that is taken in and exhaled is usually half a litre or 500 cm³ with each breath. This is known as the tidal volume. In a healthy adult approximately 70% of the tidal volume enters the alveoli, the remaining 30% remaining in the bronchial tree. Air that remains in the bronchial tree cannot be used in gas exchange and these conducting airways are known as the anatomic dead space.

The apparatus used to measure respiratory rate and the volume of air that a person inhales and exhales during breathing is called a spirometer and the results are recorded as a graph called a spirogram. A spirometer has a hollow drum over a chamber of water. As a person inhales and exhales through the mouthpiece the drum will rise and fall and the movement is recorded on a rotating chart called a spirogram.

Spirometer and spirogram

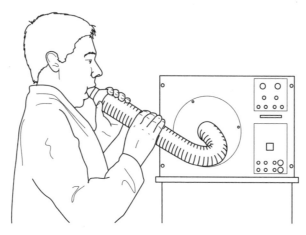

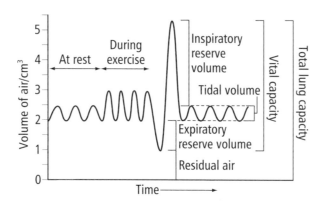

If you take a deep breath, the volume of inhaled air increases to approximately 3000 ml. This volume of air is called the inspiratory reserve volume.

If you exhale as forcibly as you can, you should be able to force out an additional 1200 ml of air as well as the 500 ml of tidal volume. The extra air pushed out is called the expiratory reserve volume. The air remaining in the lungs (approximately 1000 ml) is called the residual volume.

The ventilation rate to show the volume of air breathed per minute is calculated by multiplying tidal volume by number of inspirations. The ventilation rate will change in response to the needs of the body; for example, the ventilation rate will be higher during periods of exercise. The ventilation rate is controlled by the respiratory centre of the brain.

The respiratory centre

Control of breathing

The respiratory centre is situated in the medulla oblongata and pons varolii of the brain stem.

The respiratory centre

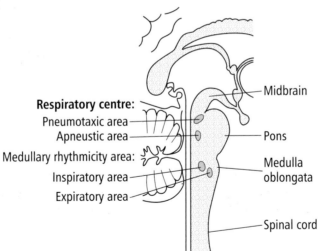

The respiratory centre determines the rhythm of respiration in response to the level of carbon dioxide in the blood.

If carbon dioxide levels rise the respiratory centre is responsible for sending nerve impulses down the phrenic nerves to the diaphragm and down the thoracic nerves to the intercostal muscles to initiate an intake of air (inspiration).

When oxygen levels in the blood drop, the respiratory centre will respond by increasing the rate and depth of breathing.

Control of respiratory movements

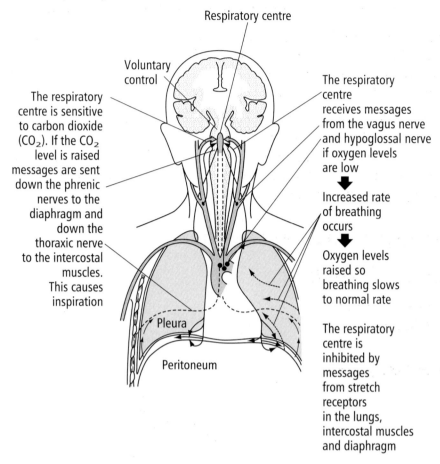

Respiratory centre

Voluntary control

The respiratory centre is sensitive to carbon dioxide (CO_2). If the CO_2 level is raised messages are sent down the phrenic nerves to the diaphragm and down the thoracic nerve to the intercostal muscles. This causes inspiration

Pleura

Peritoneum

The respiratory centre receives messages from the vagus nerve and hypoglossal nerve if oxygen levels are low

Increased rate of breathing occurs

Oxygen levels raised so breathing slows to normal rate

The respiratory centre is inhibited by messages from stretch receptors in the lungs, intercostal muscles and diaphragm

Internal respiration

Internal respiration occurs between the capillaries, the interstitial fluid and tissue cells. Internal respiration occurs throughout the body allowing the exchange of oxygen and CO_2 in tissues by means of diffusion.

4 Diseases and disorders of the respiratory system

Bronchitis

Bronchitis is a disease in which the bronchi are inflamed. Mucous builds up in the bronchi causing a productive cough. In acute bronchitis the inflammation is caused by inhaled irritants or following viral infection. The inflammation lasts for a short period of time. In chronic bronchitis the inflammation occurs on a regular basis causing long-term illness. The bronchi may become narrow and inspiration becomes more difficult. Smokers are at high risk of suffering from chronic bronchitis and the disease is progressive. The excessive secretions produced lead to obstruction of the bronchi and this predisposes the development of emphysema.

Chronic obstructive pulmonary disease (COPD)

This condition is a combination of chronic bronchitis and emphysema. Predisposing factors include smoking and/or air pollution. Excessive mucous secretions cause a constant cough in an attempt to clear the airways. Ventilation is poor causing breathlessness during exertion. Clients are prone to infection of the respiratory tract as the collection of mucous acts as a culture medium for bacteria. As the disease progresses the client will become short of breath at the slightest effort and oxygen therapy will be required.

Emphysema

In this condition the alveoli are gradually destroyed, leading to inadequate ventilation. Emphysema may be caused by chronic bronchitis or dust particles. In babies it is associated with a congenital defect of the bronchial walls.

Pleurisy

Pleurisy is an inflammation of the pleura. Causes include lung infections, lung cancer and rheumatoid arthritis. If fluid collects between the layers of the pleura, a pleural effusion will develop making inspiration difficult and painful.

Rhinitis

Rhinitis is the inflammation of the mucous membrane lining of the nose causing nasal discharge and sneezing. The cause may be viral or allergy related.

Further reading

Acheson, Sir D. (1998) *Report of the Independent Inquiry into Inequalities in Health*. The Stationery Office Ltd, London.

Department of Health (1998) *Our Healthier Nation: A Contract for Health*. The Stationery Office Ltd, London.

Ford, S. and Richardson, A. (1995) *GNVQ Human Physiology and Health in the Caring Context*. Nelson Thornes, Cheltenham.

Taylor, C., Lillis, C. and LeMone, P. (1997) *Fundamentals of Nursing: The Art and Science of Nursing Care*, 3rd edn. Nelson Thornes, Cheltenham.

Chapter 6

The digestive system

National unit specification
These are the topics you will be studying for this unit.

1 Anatomy and Physiology of the gastrointestinal tract

2 The mouth

3 The oesophagus and the stomach

4 The small intestines

5 The liver

6 The pancreas

7 The large intestines

8 Disorders of the gastrointestinal tract

Diagrams to practise

Position of organs in the digestive system

Oral cavity

Stomach

Duodenum with associated ducts from the pancreas and liver

Liver cells

Large bowel

Your assessment may include a time-constraint examination and a written report based on a practical investigation.

You may be required to demonstrate knowledge of the basic anatomy and functions of the digestive tract, including the process of digestion and relevance to healthcare.

Homeostasis

The digestive system comprises two groups of organs: the gastrointestinal tract – a tube that runs from the mouth to the anus, and the accessory organs for digestion – salivary glands, teeth, tongue, liver, gall bladder and pancreas. The digestive system breaks down food into small molecules so that the nutrients can enter the blood and lymph system.

Skin:
Small intestines absorb vitamin D.
Excess food/energy is stored in adipose cells
in the subcutaneous layer of the skin.

Skeletal system:
Calcium is absorbed by the small Intestines.

Muscular:
The liver converts lactic acid to glucose used during exercise.

Lymphatic system:
Acid in the stomach destroys bacteria and toxins.

Reproductive organs:
Provide nutrients for fetal growth and
development.

Urinary system:
Water absorbed is needed to produce urine
for excretion of waste products.

Nervous system:
Provides glucose for neurons.

Respiratory system:
Abdominal organs may be used to apply pressure
against the diaphragm to aid forcing air out of
the lungs.

Endocrine system:
Liver helps to regulate hormone activity and
the pancreas produces insulin and glucogen.

Cardiovascular system:
Water is absorbed to maintain blood volume.
Plasma protein is made by the liver.
Iron is absorbed for red blood cells.
Old red cells are made into bilirubin and excreted
in bile.

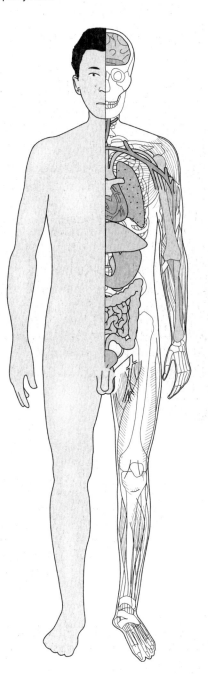

1 Anatomy and physiology of the gastrointestinal tract

We require food to ensure the growth, repair and normal function of our body systems. Food provides the body with energy and materials necessary for homeostasis. The food may be found from plant, animal and inorganic sources. Humans are classed as heterotrophic as they obtain the carbon compounds necessary for energy and growth from ingested food.

All foodstuffs are derived from organisms that harness light energy to produce biochemical molecules (autotrophic organisms). Therefore, the chemical energy required for our survival comes ultimately from the sun.

Feelings of hunger prompt us to find food. Humans have a natural mechanism to seek food and the nervous, sensory and muscular systems have evolved to help us obtain sufficient quantities of food and protect against ingestion (eating) of an array of harmful substances.

Feelings of hunger and feeling 'full up' are controlled by the hypothalamus gland. The hunger centre is active at all times except when there is input from the satiety centre – which stops us wanting to eat. There are many theories about what factor regulates food intake, but no one theory has fully explained the regulation of food intake.

When food is consumed (eaten) it has to be broken down into a form that can be used by the cells. The digestive system is designed to convert food ready for absorption and to eliminate any substances that cannot be absorbed. There are five main processes in the human digestive system:

- Ingestion: putting food into the mouth.

- Digestion: chemical and physical breakdown of food.

- Absorption: following digestion the end product is passed into the cardiovascular and lymphatic system and distributed to the body cells.

- Assimilation: the liver breaks down worn out erythrocytes and removes useful components of haemoglobin, helping to control amino acid levels necessary for homeostasis.

- Defecation: the elimination from the body of substances that are indigestible or unabsorbed.

The digestive system is a 9 m tube with a receiving end (the mouth) and a discharging end (the anus). The tube (called the alimentary canal or gastrointestinal tract) has adjoining accessory organs (teeth, salivary glands, liver, biliary system and pancreas) to aid digestion.

The gastrointestinal tract

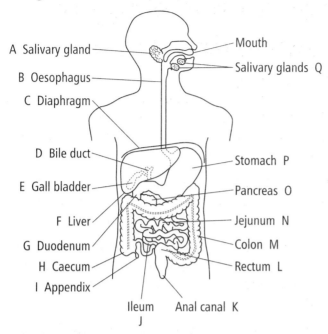

A Salivary gland
B Oesophagus
C Diaphragm
D Bile duct
E Gall bladder
F Liver
G Duodenum
H Caecum
I Appendix

Mouth
Salivary glands Q
Stomach P
Pancreas O
Jejunum N
Colon M
Rectum L

Ileum   Anal canal K
J

A	=	Green
B	=	Orange
C	=	Brown
D	=	Light blue
E	=	Pink
F	=	Red
G	=	Dark blue
H	=	Purple
I	=	Yellow
J	=	Lilac
K	=	Tan
L	=	Dark orange
M	=	Grey
N	=	Light green
O	=	Dark red
P	=	Dark pink
Q	=	Navy

* Diagram to practise

Structure of the gastrointestinal tract

The basic structure of the tube forming the GI tract remains similar throughout. The wall of the GI tract has four layers:

Structure of the wall of the GI tract

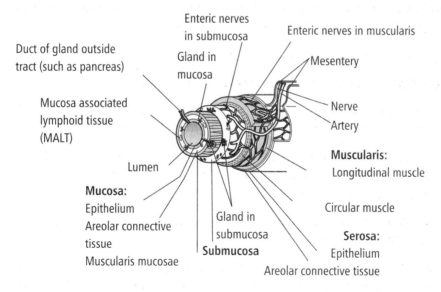

Enteric nerves in submucosa
Enteric nerves in muscularis
Duct of gland outside tract (such as pancreas)
Gland in mucosa
Mesentery
Mucosa associated lymphoid tissue (MALT)
Nerve
Artery
Lumen
Muscularis:
Longitudinal muscle
Mucosa:
Epithelium
Areolar connective tissue
Muscularis mucosae
Gland in submucosa
Circular muscle
Serosa:
Epithelium
Submucosa
Areolar connective tissue

- Mucosa: an inner lining of mucous membrane. The mucosa is made up of two layers. The inner layer secretes digestive fluids and absorbs nutrients, and the outer layer provides nutrients and defence functions for the inner layer. Mucous is secreted by simple epithelium cells and goblet cells found in columnar epithelia.

- Submucosa: this layer is made up of loose connective tissue and elastic fibres. It contains blood vessels and nerves (Meissner's plexis).

- Muscularis: in most areas this contains an outer layer of longitudinal smooth muscle and an inner layer of muscle that encircles the wall of the tube. Nerves are arranged between the muscle fibres (called Auerbach's or myenteric plexus). The parasympathetic and sympathetic nerves are responsible for coordinating contractions of the tube. The contractions of muscle occur in waves and this creates peristaltic action that pushes the contents of the tube onwards. The muscle action also helps to mix the contents with the digestive juices. There are rings of muscles called sphincters situated at various points to delay food and allow digestion and absorption to take place.

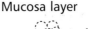
Mucosa layer

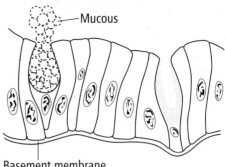
Mucous

Basement membrane

- Serosa: the outermost layer that covers all of the organs of the gastrointestinal tract. It is also known as the peritoneum (per'-i-tō-NĒ-um) and is the largest serous membrane of the body. The serosa secretes fluid to prevent friction between the organs. It forms a closed sac around the abdominal organs and has two layers:
  - Visceral peritoneum: covering the organs.
  - Parietal peritoneum or omentum (ō-MENT-um): a fold of serosa that drapes over the small intestines like an apron and contains blood, nerves and lymph vessels that supply the abdominal organs. The small intestines are attached to the posterior part of the abdominal cavity by a part of the peritoneum called the mesentery (MEZ-en-ter'-ē).

Peritoneum (shaded area)

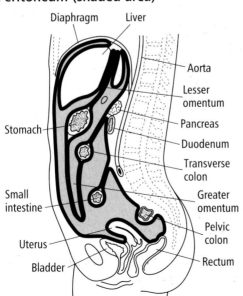

Diaphragm Liver
Aorta
Lesser omentum
Stomach
Pancreas
Duodenum
Transverse colon
Small intestine
Greater omentum
Pelvic colon
Uterus
Bladder
Rectum

The omentum

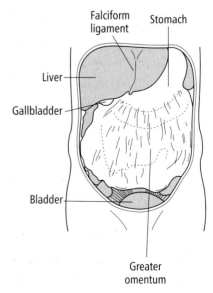

Falciform ligament Stomach
Liver
Gallbladder
Bladder
Greater omentum

2 The mouth

The mouth (oral cavity) is the entrance to the gastrointestinal tract. The mouth and associated structures begin the process of digestion by ingestion (putting food in the mouth), mastication (chewing) and production of saliva (beginning the process of chemical digestion of food).

The mouth is formed by:

- Lips.

- The muscles of the cheeks.

- Hard (bony) and soft (muscle) palates.

- The tongue.

The mouth is bound by bones of the skull and jaw.

The oral cavity

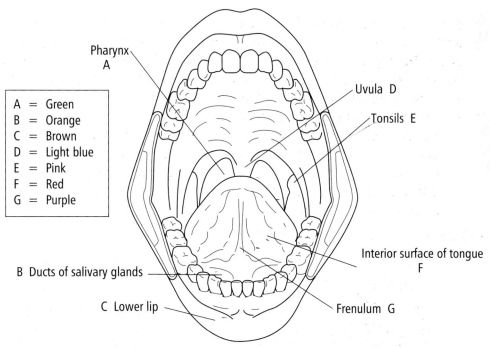

Pharynx
A

A	=	Green
B	=	Orange
C	=	Brown
D	=	Light blue
E	=	Pink
F	=	Red
G	=	Purple

Uvula D

Tonsils E

Interior surface of tongue
F

B Ducts of salivary glands

C Lower lip

Frenulum G

* Diagram to practise

The tongue

- This forms the floor of the mouth.

- It is a voluntary muscle covered by mucous membrane.

- It alters in shape and size for speech and mastication.

- The upper surface and sides are covered with papillae, small projections containing nerve endings (some containing taste buds).

- The frenulum, a fold of mucous membrane, holds the tongue to the floor of the mouth. The base or root of the tongue is attached to the hyoid bone.

- Arterial blood is supplied by the lingual branch of the external carotid artery and venous drainage is by the lingual vein that feeds into the internal jugular vein.

Taste regions of the tongue

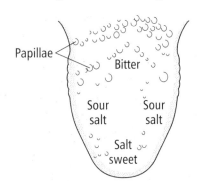

- The hypoglossal nerves supply the tongue's voluntary muscle and the mandibular nerves supply sensation. Taste buds are supplied by the facial and glossopharyngeal nerves.

The teeth

Humans have two sets of teeth. The first set, deciduous teeth, begin to appear from the age of six months and are lost between the age of six and 12 years. Permanent teeth erupt from the age of six until adulthood. There are 32 teeth in a complete set of permanent teeth.

Deciduous (milk) teeth

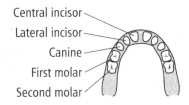

Second (permanent) teeth

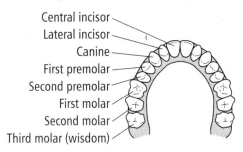

The teeth are located in the bony sockets of the mandible and maxillae. There are different teeth to perform different functions:

- Incisors: for cutting through food.

- Canines: for tearing and shredding food.

- Molars and premolars: to crush and grind food.

The structure of teeth is the same in each of the tooth types:

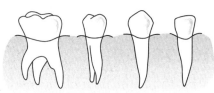

- The crown: exposed part of the tooth that extends above the gum (gingiva) – covered with enamel, a substance that is very hard and able to withstand high temperatures.

Section of a tooth

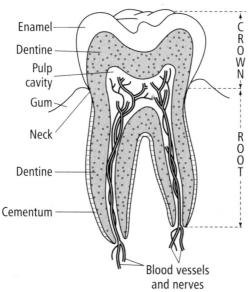

Enamel
Dentine
Pulp cavity
Gum
Neck
Dentine
Cementum

CROWN

ROOT

Blood vessels and nerves

- The neck: where the crown becomes the root.

- The root: where the tooth is embedded in bone – surrounded by a hard substance called cementum.

The inner part of the tooth is called the pulp cavity and contains the nerves, blood, and lymph vessels. Dentine is a hard substance that surrounds the pulp cavity. There is a small area at the base of the root of the tooth to allow blood and nerve vessels in and out of the tooth. The teeth are supplied with nerves from the trigeminal (fifth cranial) nerve.

Teeth aid digestion by preparing food before swallowing. Teeth also play an important role in body image and self esteem. Tooth decay and gum disease are common conditions in affluent societies. Gum disease (gingivitis) may lead to infection, loss of teeth and bone destruction.

Salivary glands

There are three pairs of salivary glands. The glands consist of numerous lobules lined with secretory cells. The glands have ducts that take the saliva into the oral cavity. The parasympathetic nerve supply stimulates secretion of saliva and the sympathetic nerves depress secretion.

Salivary glands

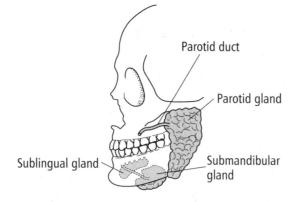

Parotid duct
Parotid gland
Sublingual gland
Submandibular gland

- The secretion of saliva aids speech, mastication, taste and swallowing.

- Saliva is made up of water (99.5%) and solvents (0.5%). The water helps to moisten and dissolve food.

- Mucous in the saliva helps to lubricate the food so that it can be swallowed more easily.

- Saliva contains an enzyme, amylase, that begins the digestion of carbohydrates.

- The enzyme lysozyme is also present and this destroys bacteria harmful to mucous membrane.

Pharynx (FĀR-inks)

Food passes into the pharynx from the mouth. This muscular area of the alimentary canal has seven openings:

- Mouth.

- Larynx.

- Two apertures from the nose.

- Two eustachian tubes from the ears.

- Oesophagus.

When a bolus (ball) of food enters the pharynx it is pushed along by peristaltic action and is no longer under voluntary control.

The swallowing reflex begins when a bolus of food is pushed into the pharynx by the tongue.

The muscles of the pharynx push (propel) the food into the oesophagus. All other openings in the pharynx are closed. The larynx is closed and covered with a flap of cartilage called the epiglottis. The epiglottis prevents food from entering the trachea. The swallowing reflex is controlled by a centre in the brain stem and involves coordinated muscle contraction of the pharynx and larynx.

The bolus of food continues down into the oesophagus (ōe-SOF-a-gus).

Swallowing (voluntary stage)

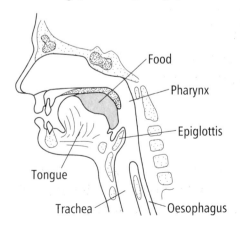

- Food
- Pharynx
- Epiglottis
- Tongue
- Trachea
- Oesophagus

Swallowing (involuntary stage)

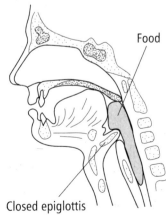

- Food
- Closed epiglottis

3 The oesophagus and the stomach

The oesophagus is a muscular tube that lies behind the trachea. Food moves down the oesophagus by peristaltic waves. The oesophagus passes through the mediastinum and diaphragm before connecting to the stomach.

The oesophagus

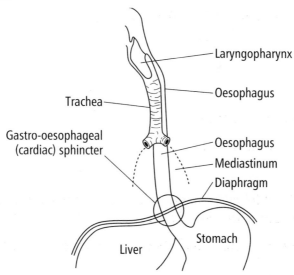

Peristaltic action

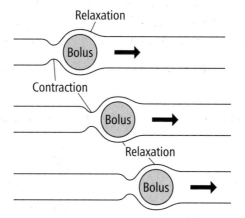

The stomach

The stomach is a widening of the gastrointestinal tract. It resembles a J-shaped bag with a capacity for approximately 2 litres of food/fluid. It is situated in the upper left abdominal cavity and is partly protected by the lower ribs.

The stomach is divided into five areas:

- Cardia (CAR-dē-a): surrounding the upper opening of the stomach.

- Fundus (FUN-dus): upper portion of the stomach that normally contains only air.

- Body: large central portion of the stomach.

- Antrum (An-t-rum): lies between the body and pyloris. It is the expanded portion of the pyloric part of the stomach.

- Pyloris (pi-LOR-us): narrow lower end of the stomach through which food leaves the stomach and enters the small intestines. Between the pyloris and small intestines there is a circular band of muscle called the pyloric sphincter. This acts as a valve to allow food to be digested in the stomach until the gastric contents are ready to enter the duodenum, the first part of the small intestines.

The stomach area has modifications to the four layered structure of its walls. The muscle fibres contain additional oblique fibres to assist in churning the food. The mucosa layer has columnar epithelia containing deep gastric pits that have gastric and mucous glands. When the stomach is empty the mucous membrane has a crumpled appearance with many folds called rugae (ROO-jē). When the stomach is full the mucous membrane is smooth. The parasympathetic nerves stimulate muscle action and gastric juice secretion.

The five areas of the stomach

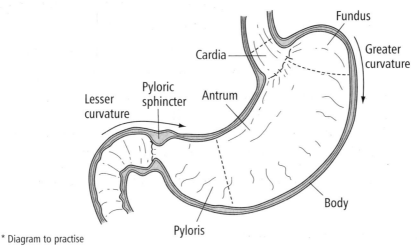

* Diagram to practise

Digestion and absorption in the stomach

As food enters the stomach mechanical digestion begins. The food is mixed as the stomach muscles begin peristaltic waves of movement. Gastric enzymes from the gastric glands are secreted and the food is churned until it becomes a thin fluid called chyme (KīM). With each peristaltic wave the chyme is pushed through the pyloric sphincter at the base of the stomach.

Gastric gland cells

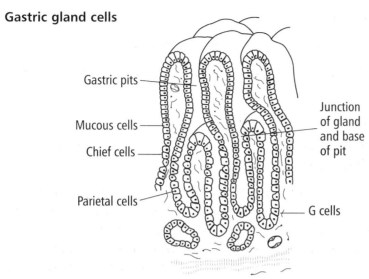

Gastric pits

Mucous cells

Chief cells

Parietal cells

Junction
of gland
and base
of pit

G cells

* Diagram to practise

Chemical digestion of food in the stomach begins when gastric juices are secreted. There are three types of gastric gland cells in the gastric pits:

- Parietal cells: producing hydrochloric acid, which acidifies the food and kills harmful microorganisms. They also produce intrinsic factor, a protein compound necessary for the absorption of vitamin B (used in the development of erythrocytes).

- Chief cells: secrete pepsinogen that produces the enzyme pepsin that begins the chemical digestion of proteins. Pepsinogen works most effectively in an acidic solution – created by the hydrochloric acid.

- G cells: secrete the hormone gastrin. This hormone stimulates muscle action of the stomach and the secretion of the gastric juices.

The mucous produced by mucous neck cells helps to form a protective barrier between the cells of the stomach wall and the acidic contents of the stomach. The mucous cells of the stomach are able to absorb a small amount of water, salts, fatty acids and lipid-soluble drugs, such as aspirin and alcohol.

The time that food is retained in the stomach will depend on the food type:

- Fatty foods: up to six hours.

- Protein based foods: up to four hours.

- Carbohydrate: up to two hours.

- Water: up to 20 minutes.

The stomach is designed to allow large quantities of food to be consumed at one time. If the stomach is surgically removed, chemical digestion will still occur in the gastrointestinal tract provided only small amounts of low-fat food are ingested.

4 The small intestines

The small intestines are divided into three segments:

- Duodenum.

- Jejunum.

- Ileum.

Each segment allows chemical digestion to continue and absorption of food to take place.

Small intestines

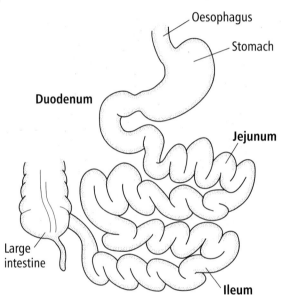

Functions

- To allow onward movement of food.

- Secretion of intestinal juices.

- Digestion of carbohydrates, fats and proteins.

- To protect the body from microorganisms by the use of lymph follicles.

- Secretion of hormones.

- Absorption of nutrients.

Structure

- The mucosa and submucosa of the small intestines are adapted for absorption of food by having fingerlike tufts called villi.

- The cells that absorb food are called microvilli (mī'-krō-VIL-ī). These cylindrical-shaped projections have an increased surface area of plasma membrane to allow for greater absorption of digested nutrients.

- There are numerous lymph nodes throughout the length of the small intestine, the larger nodules are called Peyer's patches (aggregated lymphatic follicules).

- The superior mesenteric artery and vein are responsible for the blood flow to and from the gastrointestinal tract.

- Nerve supply is from parasympathetic and sympathetic nerves.

Structure of villi

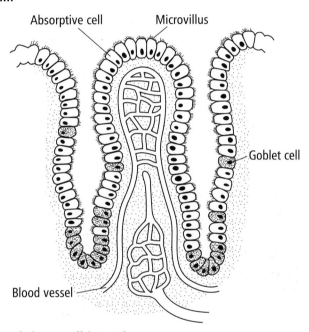

Mucosal lining of the small intestines

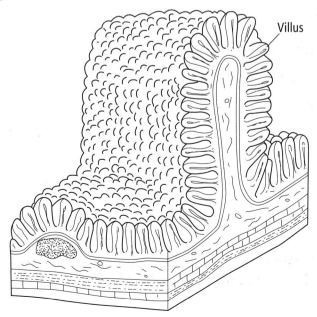

The duodenum (doo'-o-DĒ-num)

The duodenum is approximately 25 cm long and it curves around the head of the pancreas. Ducts from the pancreas and gall bladder enter at a common opening, at the midpoint of the duodenum. This opening is guarded by the sphincter of Oddi.

The chyme leaves the stomach in small amounts and enters the duodenum, the first part of the small intestines. The presence of chyme triggers the release of two hormones:

- Secretin (se-KRĒ-tin): to decrease the amount of gastric juices in the stomach.

- Cholecystokinin (kō'-lē-sis'-tō-KĪN-in): to delay or inhibit the chyme entering the duodenum.

These hormones help to regulate the food entering the duodenum to prevent food passing through too quickly. They also stimulate glands in the pancreas and liver.

Liver and related structures

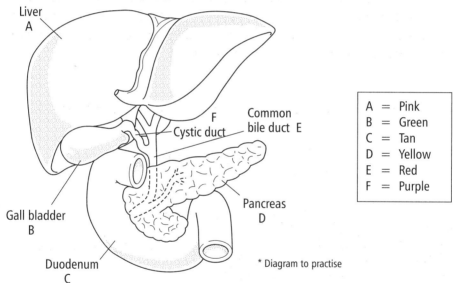

A	=	Pink
B	=	Green
C	=	Tan
D	=	Yellow
E	=	Red
F	=	Purple

* Diagram to practise

Intestinal juices

Intestinal juices found in the duodenum contain the following enzymes:

- Enterokinase: converts trypsinogen into active trypsin.

- Peptidase: acts on peptones to produce amino acids.

- Maltase: turns maltose into glucose.

- Sucrase: turns sucrose into a simple sugar such as glucose.

- Lactase: turns lactose into simple sugar.

- Lipase: completes the process of turning fats to fatty acid and glycerol.

The chyme in the duodenum is mixed with the enzymes and fluids by peristalsis and additional contractions of the intestinal muscles. Absorption of proteins, carbohydrates and fats takes place in the small intestines. Fatty acids and glycerol are absorbed by cells in the villi and enter into the lymphatic capillaries.

The Jejunum (jē-JOO-num)

The jejunum extends from the duodenum to the ileum. The jejunum is about 2.6 m long and digestion continues before food enters the final part of the small intestines.

The Ileum (IL-ē-um)

The ileum connects the small intestines with the caecum. It is approximately 3.6 m long and contains folds of epithelial membrane called villi. The villi increase the surface area to assist in the process of absorption. At the base of each villi are glands called Crypts of Lieberkuhn that secrete intestinal juice called succus entericus. This contains enzymes concerned with the chemical breakdown of food. Nutrients are absorbed at different sections of the ileum by passive diffusion, osmosis and active transport.

Jejunum and ileum showing areas where substances are digested and absorbed

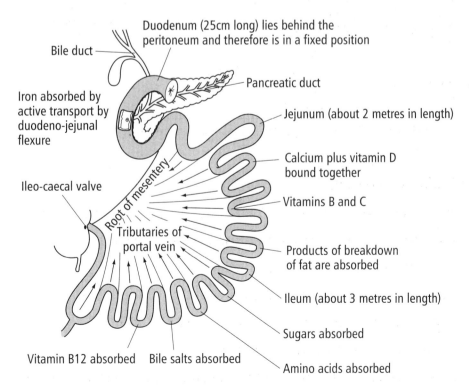

5 The liver

The liver is the largest organ in the body and weighs approximately 1.5 kg. It is an essential organ and carries out several metabolic processes necessary for the body to maintain homeostasis. It is estimated that the liver carries out over 500 functions.

The liver consists of four lobes and the gall bladder (situated in a depression on the posterior wall).

Structure of the liver

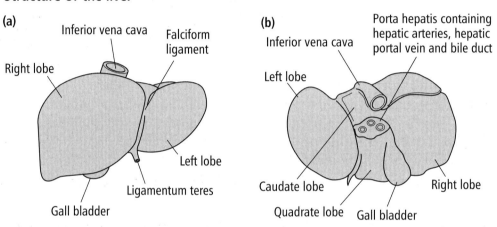

The liver is situated in the right upper abdominal cavity, protected by the rib cage. It is a very vascular organ (i.e. it has a large blood supply) and approximately 1.5 litres of blood flows through the organ each minute.

The arterial blood is received from the hepatic artery and venous blood comes from the digestive system, via the hepatic portal vein. Blood leaves the liver by the hepatic veins.

The liver is made up of lobules that are hexagonal in shape. Each lobule contains blood vessels, bile ducts, hepatocytes and Kupffer's cells.

Hepatocytes are in direct contact with blood flowing between them through venules. The hepatocytes allow chemical processes to occur in blood from the hepatic artery and the hepatic portal vein. Bile formed by the hepatocytes drains into the biliary ducts and then into the bile duct and gall bladder.

*Liver tissue

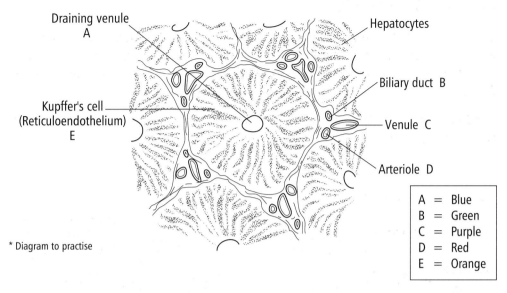

Draining venule A — Hepatocytes — Biliary duct B — Kupffer's cell (Reticuloendothelium) E — Venule C — Arteriole D

A	=	Blue
B	=	Green
C	=	Purple
D	=	Red
E	=	Orange

* Diagram to practise

Functions of the liver

- The liver produces plasma proteins including albumen and blood-clotting factors.

- It produces heparin which is a natural anticoagulant (it prevents excess clotting of the blood).

- It forms cholesterol from fat that is used for cell membranes. Excessive cholesterol is excreted by the liver in bile, but if levels are very high deposits may be found in the walls of arteries and veins. High levels of cholesterol in the bile tract and gall bladder may lead to obstruction of the common bile duct.

- The liver neutralises toxins produced by the body and from foods and drugs. This includes toxins found in the blood that is leaving the gastrointestinal tract.

- It neutralises and excretes bilirubin – the substance produced when old red blood cells are broken down. This process is carried out by specialised cells called Kupffer's cells. In high concentration, bilirubin is poisonous to body tissue.

- It regulates the level of nutrients, such as glucose, in the blood.

- It stores iron, vitamin B12, folic acid and vitamins A, D, E and K.

- To maintain homeostasis the liver is able to produce red blood cells. This only occurs in an emergency when there is a severe deficiency of red blood cells.

- The liver has a high metabolic rate and this causes it to be slightly warmer than other organs. Blood that flows through the liver is therefore warmed.

- It produces and excretes bile.

Bile

Bile is produced by the liver and stored in the gall bladder. The gall bladder is a pear-shaped sac that is attached to the liver by connective tissue. Bile is expelled by the gall bladder into the duodenum via the bile duct. Bile is an alkaline yellow/brown/green substance made by liver cells (hepatocytes) and consists of:

- Water.
- Bile salts.
- Cholesterol.
- Bile pigments.
- Salts/ions.
- Lecithin.

Flow of bile from the liver

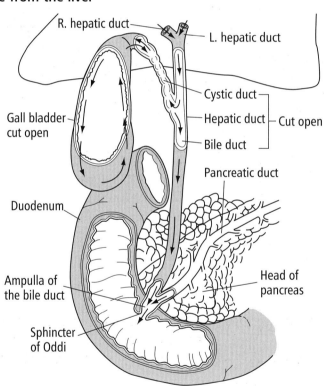

Functions of bile

- The main role of bile in the digestive process is to emulsify fatty lipids into a series of small droplets. The tiny droplets have a large surface area to allow pancreatic juices and lipase to digest them rapidly.

- Bile salts assist the absorption of digested fats, cholesterol and fat-soluble vitamins (e.g. vitamin K). Up to 90% of bile salts are reabsorbed in the lower small intestines before returning to the liver.

- Bilirubin, the principal bile pigment, gives colour to and deodorises faeces.

6 The pancreas

The pancreas is a soft pink gland that lies across the back of the abdomen behind the stomach. Its tip extends to the spleen and the rounded head fits into the curve of the duodenum. It is designed to excrete external pancreatic juice and internal insulin secretions.

Pancreas

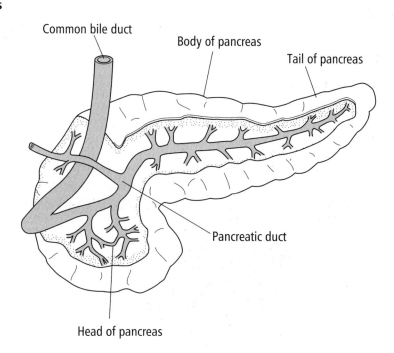

The endocrine cells are called Islets of Langerhans. Hormones from these cells are secreted directly into the bloodstream. They are a group of cells that lie between the glands which secrete the pancreatic juice. They produce the hormones:

- Glucagons: to raise blood sugar.

- Insulin: to lower blood sugar.

- Somatostatin: to maintain homeostasis by inhibiting the production of insulin and glucagons when blood glucose levels are in the normal range.

Islets of Langerhans

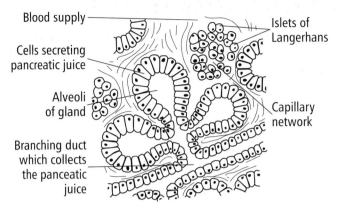

Pancreatic juice

The exocrine cells of the pancreas secrete up to 2 litres of pancreatic juice a day. These digestive juices are excreted into the pancreatic duct. The pancreatic duct and common bile duct share a single point of entry into the duodenum.

Pancreatic juice contains:

- Water.
- Mineral salts.
- Enzymes:
  - Trypsinogen: turns peptones and proteins into amino acids when it is converted into active trypsin by enterokinase which is found in the duodenum.
  - Amylase: turns starch into malt sugar (maltose).
  - Lipase: splits fat into fatty acid and glycerol following the action of bile.

7 The large intestines

The large intestines are the final part of the gastrointestinal tract, leading from the small intestines to the external skin. The large intestines are divided into the following parts:

- Caecum.
- Ascending colon.
- Transverse colon.
- Descending colon.
- Sigmoid flexure.
- The rectum.

Large intestines

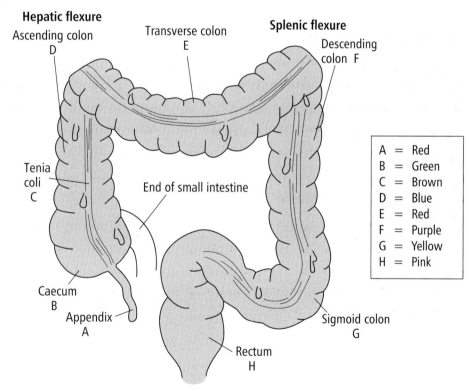

A	=	Red
B	=	Green
C	=	Brown
D	=	Blue
E	=	Red
F	=	Purple
G	=	Yellow
H	=	Pink

Function

The major functions of the large intestines are:

- Absorption of water, salt, minerals, vitamins and drugs.
- Storage of food residues, cells and bacteria until eliminated by defecation.
- Elimination of waste. When the rectum is full of faeces the sensation of pressure signals the relaxation of the sphincter muscles around the anus to allow the faeces to be expelled (defecation).

Structure

The walls of the large intestine contain the three layers that run throughout the gastrointestinal tract. There is a slight difference in the muscle layer as longitudinal muscle does not go all the way around but forms strips of muscle called tenia coli. These bands of muscle are shorter than the colon and cause puckering or haustrations.

The submucosal layer contains an abundance of lymphoid tissue to help prevent bacteria from entering the bloodstream.

Caecum

- The caecum is the first part of the large intestine (commonly referred to as the colon).

- It appears as a dilated portion of the large bowel and is situated at the junction of the small and large bowel in the lower right-hand side of the abdomen.

- There is an anatomical valve between the small and large intestine called the ileo-caecal valve which prevents backflow.

- A small, fine, blind-ended tube called the vermiform appendix leads from the caecum. The function of the appendix is not known. It contains lymph tissue but it is often a site for inflammation causing appendicitis.

Cross-section of large intestine

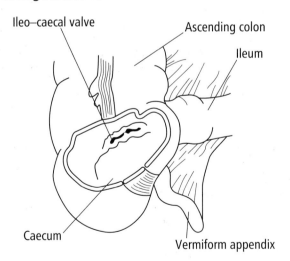

Ascending, transverse and descending colon

- The ascending colon passes upwards to the level of the liver and then turns to form the transverse colon.

- The transverse colon is a section of colon that goes across the abdomen in front of the duodenum and stomach. It bends downwards over the spleen area, called the splenic flexure, and then it becomes the descending colon.

- The descending colon is situated on the left side of the abdomen and curves in the midline of the abdomen before entering the pelvic cavity.

- The s-shaped curve of the colon before entering the pelvis is called the sigmoid colon.

Rectum

- The rectum is situated immediately in front of the sacrum.

- It forms the last 15 cm of the large intestine (3 cm in babies).

- The rectum acts as a reservoir for faeces (also called stools).

- The rectum is empty until the intervals when peristaltic action propels faeces onwards from the sigmoid colon.

- Nerve impulses from the distended rectum trigger the reflex of defecation. This reflex is inhibited until it is convenient to defecate.

Process of defecation

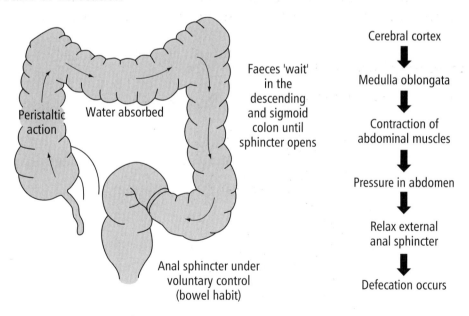

'Normal' defecation may be 3 times a day to 2-3 times a week

Anus

- The anus is a short canal that leads to the exterior. There are two sphincter muscles that control the anus.

- The internal sphincter consists of smooth muscle that is controlled by the autonomic nervous system.

- The external sphincter consists of striated muscle and is under voluntary control.

- Parasympathetic nerves cause the sigmoid colon and rectum to contract and the internal sphincter to relax.

- The pudendal nerve allows voluntary control over the external anal sphincter (from the age of 18 months onwards).

- Eating and drinking stimulate the desire to empty the bowel due to the gastro-colic reflex.

Rectum and anal canal

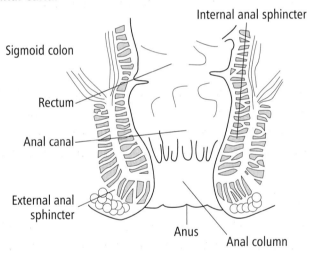

Sigmoid colon

Internal anal sphincter

Rectum

Anal canal

External anal sphincter

Anus

Anal column

8 Disorders of the gastrointestinal tract

Acute appendicitis

Appendicitis occurs when the opening into the appendix is obstructed, allowing bacteria growth within the appendix. The appendix will become inflamed and swollen leading to abdominal pain, nausea and vomiting. If left untreated the appendix may rupture spreading faecal matter within the abdominal cavity and causing inflammation of the peritoneum (peritonitis). Peritonitis is a life-threatening condition and requires immediate medical treatment.

Acute gastroenteritis

An infection of the small or large bowel caused by bacteria or virus may result in severe vomiting and diarrhoea. The infection is ingested with contaminated food and this is a common disease worldwide.

Diarrhoea

Diarrhoea is when frequent, loose or watery stools are passed. If over 300 mls of liquid faeces is lost in a 24-hour period, investigations to establish the cause are necessary. If prompt fluid replacement therapy is not given, acute diarrhoea may lead to severe fluid and electrolyte loss and eventually death.

Haemorrhoids

Haemorrhoids are varicosed or dilated veins around the anus and rectum. They are a relatively common problem in pregnant women and adults over the age of 30. If the haemorrhoids cause bleeding during defecation or severe pain and discomfort it may be necessary to remove them surgically (haemorrhoidectomy).

Peptic ulcer

Peptic ulcers are found at sites that are bathed in gastric juices. The most common sites are the stomach and duodenum. In this condition the mucosa layer breaks down causing a small area to become exposed to the acid contents of the stomach thus creating an ulcer. The cause of the ulcer is often due to bacteria, specifically Helicobacter pylori. A lifestyle that includes smoking or drinking alcohol will increase the risk of developing an ulcer and it is estimated that 10% of the population will suffer from a peptic ulcer. The ulcer may erode through blood vessels and/or the wall of the stomach/duodenum, causing a perforation that allows the gastric contents to leak into the abdominal cavity. If this occurs emergency surgery is required to control the bleeding and to suture (sew) over the hole made by the ulcer.

Tooth decay

Tooth decay or dental caries is caused by a gradual softening of the enamel and dentin of a tooth by bacterial acids formed in the mouth as starchy and sugary food decay. Microorganisms may then invade the pulp, causing inflammation and infection.

Viral hepatitis

Viruses that result in inflammation of the liver are a common cause of liver disease. The disease is usually identified by yellow discolouring of the skin (jaundice) due to a raised level of bilirubin in the plasma. Several different viruses may affect the liver, the most common ones being:

- Hepatitis A: formerly known as infective hepatitis. A viral infection caused by ingesting food contaminated by faeces of a hepatitis A sufferer. The disease is self-limiting as antibody production is quickly activated, and it often passes unnoticed in childhood. Following infection the person has a probable lifelong immunity.

- Hepatitis B: formerly known as serum hepatitis. This virus is spread by blood, secretions and sexual intercourse. The virus may remain active in the liver and over a period of years it can cause irreversible damage to the liver cells.

- Hepatitis C: similar to hepatitis B. Cirrhosis and liver cancer may develop many years after the original contact.

- Hepatitis D: hepatitis D virus has as yet only been found in people with the hepatitis B virus. The combined B and D virus increase the risk of severe liver damage.

- Hepatitis E: is spread in the same way as hepatitis A. It does not cause chronic liver damage but it is potentially fatal in women who are pregnant.

Vaccines are available against hepatitis B and immunisation programmes include vaccination of all school children in England and all National Health Service healthcare workers.

Further reading

Arnould-Taylor, W. (2001) *A Textbook of Anatomy and Physiology*, 3rd edn. Nelson Thornes, Cheltenham.

Boyle, M., Inge, B. and Senior, K. (1999) *Human Biology*. Collins Educational, London.

Fullick, A. (2000) *Biology*. Heinemann, Oxford.

Memmler, R. L., Cohen, B. J. and Wood, D. L. (1996) *Structure and Function of the Human Body*. J. B. Lippincott, Philadelphia.

Ross, J. and Wilson, K. (1985) *Foundations of Anatomy and Physiology*, 5th edn. Churchill Livingstone, London.

Vellacott, J. and Side, S. (1998) *Understanding Advanced Human Biology*. Hodder and Stoughton, London.

Chapter 7

The genital-urinary system

National unit specification
These are the topics you will be studying for this unit.

1 The urinary system

2 Diseases and disorders of the urinary system

3 The reproductive system

4 Diseases and disorders of the reproductive system

Diagrams to practise

The urinary system

A nephron

Section through the bladder

Male reproductive structures

Female reproductive structures

Ovary and follicles

The genital-urinary system includes the excretive system and the reproductive system. Although the systems may be viewed separately the organs involved are often common to both.

Homeostasis

The kidneys are vital organs and they regulate the volume and composition of fluids in the body. Waste products from the blood are excreted in urine via the bladder and urethra. If the kidneys fail (end-stage renal failure), daily dialysis or a kidney transplant is necessary to maintain homeostasis.

Skin:
Vitamin D.

Skeletal system:
Maintain levels of calcium and phosphates .

Muscular system:
Adjust calcium levels for muscle contraction.

Nervous system:
Provide glucose for neurons.

Endocrine system:
Hormones released to help with production of red blood cells.

Cardiovascular system:
Adjust blood volume and blood pressure.
Red cell breakdown converted to bilirubin.

Lymphatic system:
Adjust volume of lymph and intestinal fluid.

Urinary system:
Removes microbes from the urethra by the flow of urine.

Respiratory system:
Maintains body fluids.

Digestive system:
Activates vitamin D necessary for absorption of calcium.

Reproductive system:
In males, part of the urethra is used for expelling semen as well as urine.

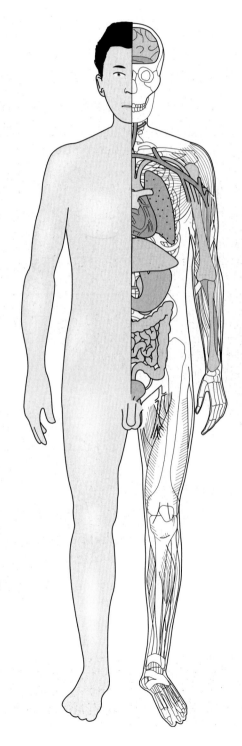

1 The urinary system

The urinary system consists of four areas:

- Two kidneys:
    - To regulate blood volume and chemical composition.
    - To help regulate blood pressure.
    - To regulate the acid-base balance of blood.

- Two ureters:
    - Transport urine from the kidneys to the urinary bladder.
    - Urinary bladder:
    - Stores urine until the need to expel via the urethra.

- Urethra:
    - Urine is discharged from the body through the urethra.

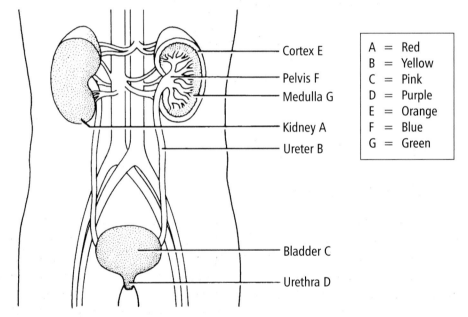

Cortex E
Pelvis F
Medulla G
Kidney A
Ureter B
Bladder C
Urethra D

A = Red
B = Yellow
C = Pink
D = Purple
E = Orange
F = Blue
G = Green

* Diagram to practise

The kidneys are responsible for the main functions of the urinary system. The most important function is to maintain homeostasis by regulating the chemical composition and volume of body fluids.

The body requires nutrients in order to maintain homeostasis. The process of delivering the nutrients includes many chemical reactions that are referred to as metabolism. The metabolic reactions produce nutrients and also waste products. The waste products may be harmful or toxic to the body and must be removed or excreted.

Excretion is the removal of substances that are derived from body fluids and occurs in faeces, sweat, expired gases and the kidneys. The kidneys are the main organs of excretion.

The kidneys

The kidneys are a pair of organs that are situated in the abdominal cavity. They are outside the peritoneum on either side of the spinal column with the right kidney slightly lower than the left. Each kidney is a bean-shaped organ approximately 12 cm long, enclosed in the renal capsule (fibrous membrane) and embedded in fatty (adipose) tissue.

Blood is supplied to the kidney by the renal artery and the nerve supply is from branches of the autonomic nervous system. The renal vein transports blood away from the kidney. The vessels enter and leave the kidney from an area called the renal hilus or hilum.

Renal vessels and nerves

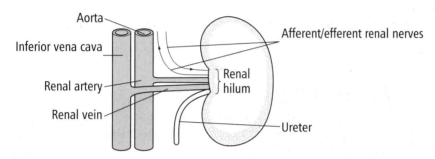

Functions of the kidneys

Regulation of blood volume

The volume of water in the circulatory system must be kept constant to maintain homeostasis. The amount of water ingested varies considerably and if large volumes are taken in, the kidneys will excrete large amounts of pale diluted urine. If fluid intake is low the kidneys will excrete small amounts of concentrated urine. Fluid balance is measured by observing the intake (positive balance) of fluid and the output (negative balance) of urine. The difference observed in balances over a 24-hour period should remain minimal if kidney function is effective.

Regulation of blood pressure

The kidneys help to regulate blood pressure by adjusting blood volume and secreting the hormone renin that will lead to the kidneys reabsorbing more water.

Regulation of electrolytes

The concentration levels of ions including sodium, potassium, calcium, chloride and phosphates (collectively termed electrolytes) must be kept within limits necessary for homeostasis. A minor increase or decrease deviating from normal limits will have significant consequences – in some cases fatal. The kidneys help to regulate and maintain normal blood concentrations of electrolytes.

Excretion of waste products

By producing urine, substances that are no longer useful (e.g. toxins and drugs) are excreted through the kidneys.

Hormone production

The hormones produced by the kidney are:

- Erythropoietin (e-rith′-rō-POY-ē-tin): released to promote production of red blood cells when low oxygen levels are detected.

- Renin: if blood pressure falls in the renal artery the kidney produces the hormone renin to stimulate secretion of hormones to cause vasoconstriction in order to raise blood pressure. Renin also promotes secretion of the hormone aldosterone which decreases water and electrolyte loss from the kidneys. The increase in blood volume raises the blood pressure.

- Vitamin D: produced by the skin, liver and kidney. The active form of Vitamin D is calcitriol and this is necessary for the regulation of calcium and phosphorous stores; it is also important in the mineralisation of bones.

Internal anatomy of the kidney

A kidney consists of a solid section containing minute tubules and a cavity called the pelvis.

- The outer surface is covered with a capsule made of connective tissue.

- The outer part of the kidney is the renal cortex. The cortex is very vascular and it contains minute twisted tubules called nephrons.

- The middle part is called the renal medulla. Within the medulla are straight collecting tubules that form a number of cone-shaped structures called renal pyramids.

- The tip of the renal pyramid projects via fine tubes into the minor calyx and then the major calyces leading to the renal pelvis.

- The funnel-shaped renal pelvis receives urine that will drain into the ureter to be collected in the bladder.

Anatomy of the kidney

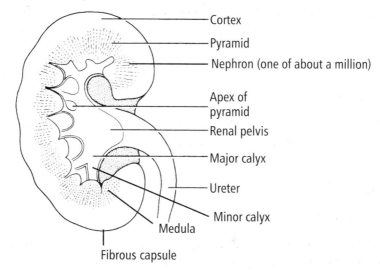

Cortex
Pyramid
Nephron (one of about a million)
Apex of pyramid
Renal pelvis
Major calyx
Ureter
Minor calyx
Medula
Fibrous capsule

Urine formation

Urine formation is a complicated process.

- The process begins with blood plasma being filtered as it passes through the kidney.

- The composition of the fluid filtered is similar to plasma and it contains glucose, amino acids, salts, urea and uric acid. Plasma proteins and blood cells are too large to be filtered in a healthy kidney.

- Large volumes of fluid are filtered, approximately 160 litres per day. The filtering units are called glomerulus.

- Reabsorption of substances needed for homeostasis occurs. All glucose is reabsorbed unless disease is present. Remaining fluid is used to produce urine.

- Secretions of substances actively occurs in the tubules. This will regulate the final composition of urine. Urine contains substances including urea and hydrogen ions that help to eliminate acids from the bloodstream.

- Regulation of body fluid is controlled by the secretion of anti-diuretic hormone (ADH) from the posterior lobe of the pituitary gland. Reabsorption of salts is controlled by hormones of the adrenal cortex.

Nephron

The nephron (NEF-ron) is the functional unit of the kidney. There are approximately one million nephrons in each kidney.

Structure of a nephron

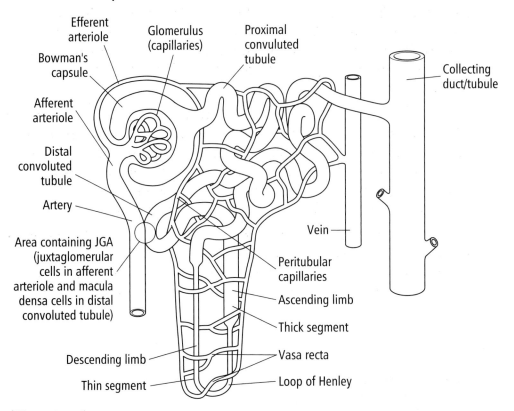

Efferent arteriole

Glomerulus (capillaries)

Proximal convoluted tubule

Collecting duct/tubule

Bowman's capsule

Afferent arteriole

Distal convoluted tubule

Artery

Area containing JGA (juxtaglomerular cells in afferent arteriole and macula densa cells in distal convoluted tubule)

Vein

Peritubular capillaries

Ascending limb

Thick segment

Descending limb

Vasa recta

Thin segment

Loop of Henley

* Diagram to practise

- A nephron consists of two parts: the renal corpuscle to filter blood plasma and a renal tubule to transport filtered fluid.

- In each nephron an arteriole enters the capsule where it becomes coiled before exiting the capsule. The capsule and coiled arteriole are the capillary network called a glomerulus.

- The capsule has a double-walled epithelial layer that has a capsular space between the layers.

- The arteriole in the glomerulus is semipermeable to allow small molecules to pass through its wall and enter the space within the glomerular (Bowman's) capsule.

Glomerular (Bowman's) capsule

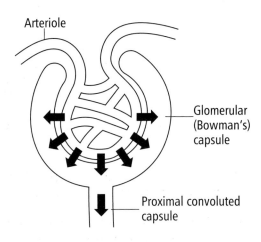

Arteriole

Glomerular (Bowman's) capsule

Proximal convoluted capsule

- Glomerular filtrate passes into the first part of the tubule called the proximal convoluted tubule. The convoluted part enlarges the surface area to increase the contact between capillaries and the tubule. This allows nutrients to be reabsorbed. Approximately two-thirds of water and sodium ions are reabsorbed here.

- Filtrate then enters the loop of Henley where reabsorption of water and solutes continues. The loop of Henley dips down into the medulla of the kidney to the point of the renal pyramid. Sodium is taken from the filtrate from the ascending limb of the loop into the descending limb. This raises the salt level in the apex of the renal pyramids. As fluid flows through the tubules, water will be reabsorbed by osmosis (high sodium levels attract water).

- The distal end of the loop is convoluted tubule. This section of the tubule has an area containing juxtaglomerular cells that are sensitive to the blood pressure of the arteriole and help to regulate filtration and blood pressure. The distal convoluted tubules of several nephrons empty into a single collecting duct.

Selective reabsorption

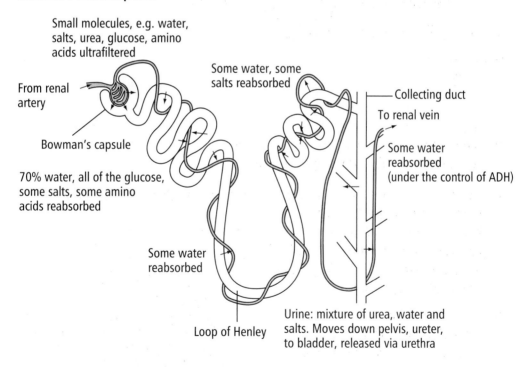

Small molecules, e.g. water, salts, urea, glucose, amino acids ultrafiltered

Some water, some salts reabsorbed

From renal artery

Collecting duct

To renal vein

Bowman's capsule

Some water reabsorbed (under the control of ADH)

70% water, all of the glucose, some salts, some amino acids reabsorbed

Some water reabsorbed

Loop of Henley

Urine: mixture of urea, water and salts. Moves down pelvis, ureter, to bladder, released via urethra

- Selective reabsorption ensures that nutritionally important substances are reabsorbed in order to maintain the body's fluid and salt balance.

- Anti-diuretic hormone affects the permeability of the distal convoluted tubule. If concentrations of salts are high, more ADH will be produced. The walls of the distal tubule will then become more permeable to allow more water to be absorbed in order to balance blood concentration. If ADH is deficient, water reabsorption is reduced, urine output is high and this may lead to dehydration – a condition that indicates diabetes insipidus.

- The collecting ducts unite in the renal pyramids. The ducts drain into the minor calyces and on into the major calyces.

Composition of urine

Urine is formed by filtration in the capsule, reabsorption and secretion in the tubules. Healthy adults produce an average of 1.5 litres each day, depending on fluid intake, diet, environmental conditions and activity.

Urine is an amber-coloured fluid. The more concentrated the urine the darker the colour. It is acid in reaction and has a characteristic odour. The odour becomes much stronger if an infection is present.

Urine is 96% water and 4% solids. The solid material consists of:

- Urea and creatinine (from muscle).

- Salts including sodium, ammonium and potassium.
- Drug and hormone waste.

Ureters

The ureters convey urine from the renal pelvis to the bladder. They are approximately 25 cm long and enter the bladder through the posterior wall.

The ureters are formed from three basic layers of connective tissue, smooth muscle and epithelial mucosa. The muscle produces a peri-

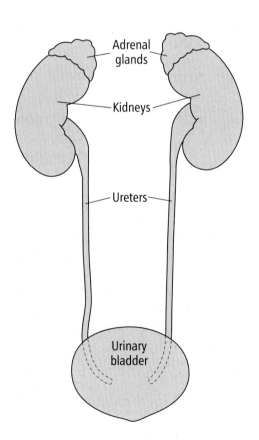

staltic action that propels the urine into the bladder. If any solid particles, such as a blood clot, are in the urine the muscle will go into spasm and cause severe pain (renal colic).

Bladder

The bladder is a muscular bag that acts as a temporary storage reservoir for urine. It lies behind the symphysis pubis when empty. When the bladder is full the upper part rises into the abdomen. The shape and size of the bladder varies according to its content. Both ureters and the urethra enter the bladder at the base approximately 3 cm from each other. This area is called the trigone. The ureters enter at an oblique angle and when the bladder contracts the muscle of the bladder wall closes the openings to prevent backflow. To prevent leakage of urine a sphincter muscle encircles the exit opening into the urethra.

The wall of the bladder consists of four layers:

- Peritoneum: the upper surface of the bladder is covered with peritoneum. This surface area is in contact with coils of small bowel. The remaining outer covering consists of fibrous tissue.

- Smooth muscle layer: the detrusor muscle. This muscle thickens at the bladder–urethral junction to form the internal urethral sphincter. Involuntary contraction of the muscle opens the sphincter and allows urine into the urethra.

- Submucosa layer: containing connective tissue, blood vessels and nerves.

- Transitional epithelium: lines the bladder in folds/rugae to allow the bladder to distend.

Position of bladder in males and females

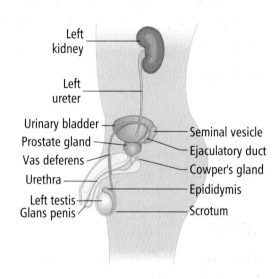

Left kidney
Left ureter
Urinary bladder
Prostate gland
Vas deferens
Urethra
Left testis
Glans penis
Seminal vesicle
Ejaculatory duct
Cowper's gland
Epididymis
Scrotum

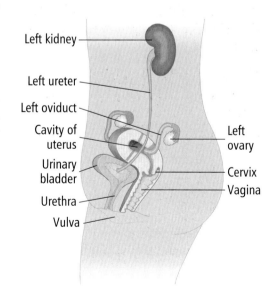

Left kidney
Left ureter
Left oviduct
Cavity of uterus
Urinary bladder
Urethra
Vulva
Left ovary
Cervix
Vagina

The bladder stores urine until micturition (the passing of urine).

The sensation of a full bladder causes the desire to pass urine. The internal urethral sphincter remains closed until it is convenient to pass urine (in babies and infants this is a reflex action). Impulses from the cortex area of the brain pass down the spinal cord to the sacral segments, along the parasympathetic nerves to stimulate the detrusor muscle to contract – this opens the internal sphincter. At the same time voluntary relaxation of the perineal muscles and the external sphincter occurs. The diaphragm and abdominal muscles contract to raise

Interior view of bladder

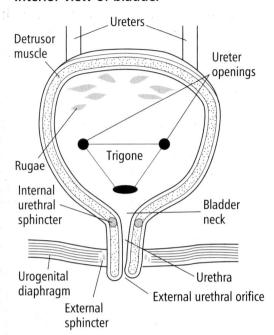

* Diagram to practise

Nerve control of micturition

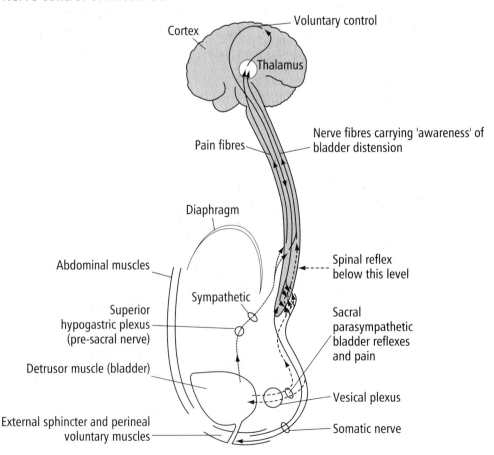

interabdominal pressure and the bladder empties. If the urge to pass urine is ignored the cerebral cortex will inhibit the detrusor muscle and the bladder will enlarge to continue to fill with urine. The desire to micturate may go away for a time, but eventually the internal sphincter will relax to relieve the pressure.

Urethra

The urethra conveys urine from the bladder to the outside skin.

The female urethra is approximately 4 cm long and opens externally in the vulva, anterior to the vaginal orifice.

The male urethra is approximately 20 cm long and it runs in a curved course

Male and female urethra

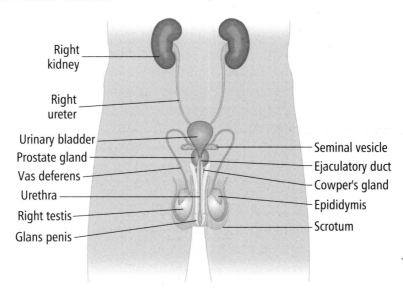

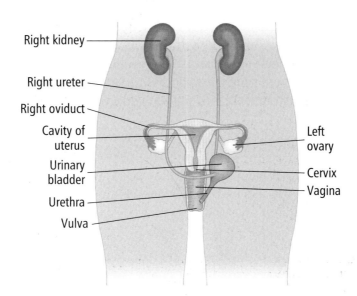

through the prostate gland, connective tissue and the penis. The male urethra has dual excretory and reproductive functions and is the common passage for urine and the ejaculation of semen.

The urethra has a further urethral sphincter formed by skeletal muscle at the pelvic floor. This external sphincter is under voluntary control.

2 Diseases and disorders of the urinary system

Acute cystitis

The bladder and urethra are resistant to infection because of the sphincters and because of the frequent flushing of urine. Acute cystitis is an inflammation of the mucosa. Cystitis is more common in women due to the shortness of the urethra. The infection that causes the inflammation may be introduced by: infection from outside (especially if a urinary catheter is introduced), urethral infection, renal infection, or if trauma occurs. Factors that predispose cystitis include retention of urine (obstruction), infection, pregnancy and diabetes mellitus. Bacteria, chemical irritants (lead, mercury, arsenic etc.), mechanical irritants (foreign bodies, catheters), parasites and fungi are all agents that may cause cystitis.

In women there may be an absence of readily identifiable bacteria and the cause may remain unknown. The condition may be induced by stress, sexual intercourse, nylon underwear or cold weather.

Acute renal failure

Renal failure is the term used when there is a decrease in glomerular filtration. The cause may be due to shock, dehydration, heart failure, infection, high calcium levels or obstruction of urine outflow. The reduced urine output will result in raised levels of urea, creatinine and potassium in the blood. Emergency treatment is required to restore fluid and salt ions (electrolyte) balance.

Calculi

Urinary calculi are stones composed of urinary salts. They may form in the kidney and bladder, but they are also found in the ureter and urethra. The cause of stone formation is unknown but several factors may be contributory, for example:

- Urine infection.
- High calcium levels.

- Vitamin A deficiency.

- Alkaline urine: caused by diet.

Stones may differ in size, shape and colour. Small stones are the commonest, but large calculi may form in the pelvis of the kidney (stag-horn calculi).

The stone or stones may cause obstruction, ulceration, haematuria or infection.

Glomerulonephritis

The glomeruli may become inflamed. A common cause of the inflammation is the toxins produced by streptococcal bacteria. If the glomeruli become swollen the filtration membranes will allow blood cells and plasma proteins to pass through and this will result in the presence of blood (haematuria) and protein in the urine.

3 The reproductive system

Human reproduction is essential for the survival of the species. Homeostatic controls such as decreased fertility during famine, reduction or loss of cellular function as a result of the ageing process, and death are factors that are essential to species' continuity but they have minimal effect, if any, on the maintenance of the homeostatic balance of the human body.

The basic purpose of men and women is to reproduce, but their functional roles are very different. Apart from the physical aspect, humans have complex psychological and sociological behaviours that influence sexual behaviour and sexuality not linked to reproduction. The reproductive organs are not functional until the onset of puberty. The male system remains functional from puberty throughout life and the reproductive role starts and ends with intercourse. The female system remains functional only until menopause, but the reproductive role extends from intercourse to childbirth.

The male reproductive system

Functions

The main functions of the male reproductive system are:

- Production of male gametes (spermatozoa).

- Transport of sperm to the female reproductive tract.

- Production of the male sex hormone (tesosterone), which controls the development of the secondary sexual characteristics (development of male physique, body, pubic and facial hair).

Sagittal section of the male reproductive system

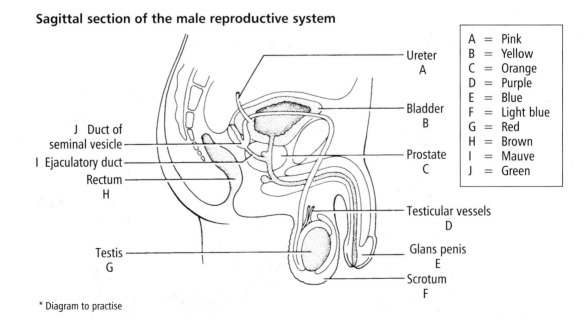

A	= Pink
B	= Yellow
C	= Orange
D	= Purple
E	= Blue
F	= Light blue
G	= Red
H	= Brown
I	= Mauve
J	= Green

Ureter A
Bladder B
Prostate C
Testicular vessels D
Glans penis E
Scrotum F

J Duct of seminal vesicle
I Ejaculatory duct
Rectum H
Testis G

* Diagram to practise

The male reproductive system consists of:

- Left and right testes and epididymis.
- The deferent ducts.
- The seminal vesicles.
- The ejaculatory ducts.
- The prostate gland.
- The penis and urethra.

The scrotum

The scrotum (SKRŌ-tum) is a pouch of loose skin and smooth muscle containing the testes. A septum divides the scrotum internally for the left and right testes. The scrotum is located outside the body as sperm need to be cooler than the normal body temperature in order to be produced and survive. Muscle fibres help to maintain temperature control by contracting (to elevate the testes in cold weather) and relaxing in warm conditions (to lower the testes and increase the surface area of the scrotum).

Testes

The testes (TES-tēz) or testicles are the glands that produce the male reproductive cells, the spermatozoa (sper-ma'-tō-ZO-a).

The testis (singular) is surrounded by connective tissue that divides it into approximately 200 lobules. In each lobule there are one to three tiny tubules called seminiferous tubules that produce sperm by the process of cell division. The process of the production of sperm is called spermatogenesis and this continues throughout life.

The testis and spermatic cord   **Structure of the testis**

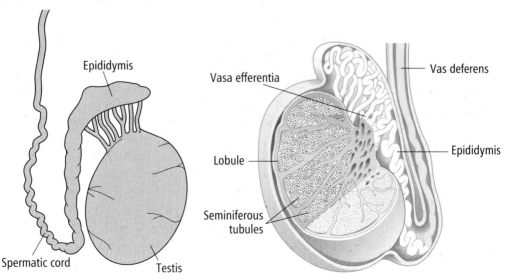

Sperm are produced in the walls of the seminiferous tubules by division and differentiation of primordial sex cells. The process takes approximately 72 days. Stem cells are positioned towards the outside of the tubules and they mature as they progress to the lumen. The mature sperm is released into the tubule for transport to the outside of the testis for further maturation.

Section of a seminiferous tubule

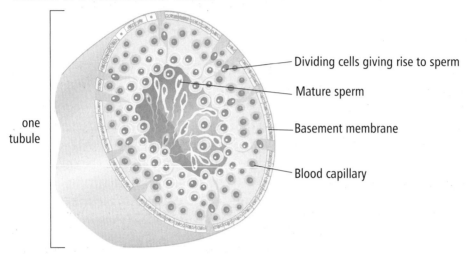

one tubule

Dividing cells giving rise to sperm

Mature sperm

Basement membrane

Blood capillary

Sertoli cells are located between sperm cells in the seminiferous tubules. These cells protect and nourish the spermatogenic cells, secrete fluid for sperm transport and also release the hormone inhibin to help regulate sperm production. Leydig (interstitial) cells are found between the seminiferous tubules and they are responsible for the secretion of testosterone.

Structure of a sperm cell

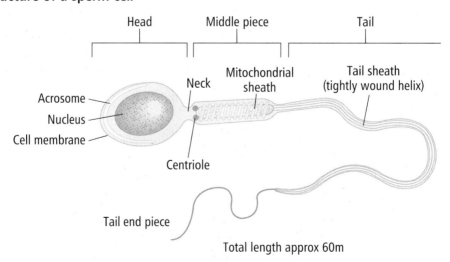

Head　　　Middle piece　　　Tail

Neck

Mitochondrial sheath

Tail sheath (tightly wound helix)

Acrosome

Nucleus

Cell membrane

Centriole

Tail end piece

Total length approx 60m

The sperm cells comprise a head, mid-piece and a tail. The mid-piece section acts like a motor to make the tail spin and propel the sperm. The head contains genetic material in the form of chromosomes and it is covered with a sheath containing digestive enzymes needed to penetrate the wall of the female ovum. There are 23 single chromosomes in the mature sperm including a male sex chromosome (Y) or a female sex chromosome (X).

Epididymis

The convoluted seminiferous tubules lead into straight tubules. The straight tubules ascend and join together to form the efferent ducts. The efferent ducts lead into a convoluted tubule called the epididymis. The epididymis sits on top of the testis and can be felt through the scrotum. The sperm undergo further maturation in the epididymis and after 14 days the sperm acquire the ability to move.

Spermatic cord

The mature sperm enter the spermatic cord (vas deferens) propelled by smooth muscle (rapid contractions convey mature sperm into the urethra during ejaculation). The spermatic cord passes into the abdominal cavity through the inguinal canal. The two spermatic cords pass above and behind the urinary bladder before entering the prostate gland to join the urethra.

The seminal vesicles

The seminal vesicles are glands situated on the posterior wall of the urinary bladder. They each have an ejaculatory duct that enters the prostate gland. The seminal vesicles are lined with epithelium that produces a viscous alkaline fluid containing glucose to nourish the sperm, amino acids, ascorbic acid, clotting enzymes and prostaglandins. This fluid forms most of the volume of semen, the fluid that is produced at ejaculation.

Prostate gland

The first part of the male urethra is surrounded by the prostate gland. This structure consists of several glands enclosed within a capsule. Within the prostate gland the ejaculatory duct joins the urethra. The prostate gland secretes a thin milky substance containing chemicals and enzymes that are needed by the sperm to help with mobility and modification of vaginal acidity. This is added to semen during ejaculation.

Posterior view of the prostate gland

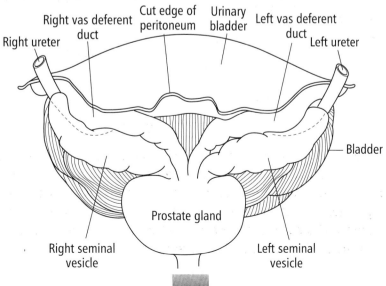

Bulbourethral glands (Cowper's glands)

Cowper's glands are tiny glands located below the prostate. They secrete a small amount of lubricating mucous into the urethra before ejaculation. This fluid lubricates the tip of the penis prior to intercourse and it neutralises the acid environment of the urethra.

Penis

The urethra passes through the prostate and down the centre of the penis. The penis is composed of spongy erectile tissue that is arranged in three columns. The urethra runs through one column to the urinary meatus. The columns begin in the pelvis (root of the penis) and run up to the enlarged tip of the penis, called the glans penis. The prepuce (PRĒ-pyoos), also called the foreskin, is a loose double fold of skin that covers the glans.

The spongy erectile tissue contain vascular spaces that fill with blood. During sexual excitement the arteries dilate to allow additional blood flow to the erectile tissue. The veins constrict trapping the blood within the erectile tissue

Internal structure of the penis

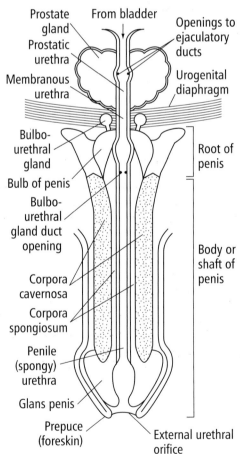

columns. This causes the penis to become enlarged and rigid. The constriction and dilatation of vessels is due to a parasympathetic reflex.

Ejaculation is a sympathetic reflex. This reflex closes the internal bladder sphincter to stop urine being expelled during ejaculation and to prohibit semen entering the bladder.

Female reproductive system

The female reproductive system consists of:

- The external genitalia, collectively called the vulva:
  - The mons pubis.
  - The labia majora.
  - The perineum.
  - The labia minora.
  - The clitoris.
  - The vestibule.
  - Orifice of the urethra.
  - Orifice of the vagina.
  - Fossa navicularis.
  - The greater vestibular glands.

- The internal reproductive organs:
  - The vagina.
  - The uterus.
  - Two fallopian tubes.
  - Two ovaries.

Sagittal section of the female organs of reproduction

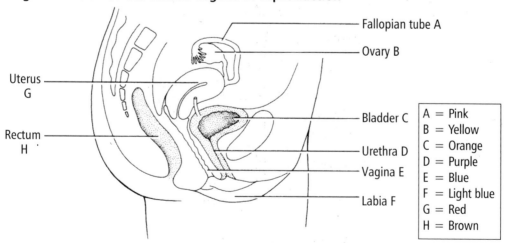

A	= Pink
B	= Yellow
C	= Orange
D	= Purple
E	= Blue
F	= Light blue
G	= Red
H	= Brown

Fallopian tube A
Ovary B
Uterus G
Rectum H
Bladder C
Urethra D
Vagina E
Labia F

* Diagram to practise

External genitalia

The vulva

The mons pubis (MONZ PYOO-bis) is a pad of fat covered with skin and, after puberty, pubic hair. From the mons pubis, two folds of fatty tissue covered with skin called the labia majora (LĀ-bēa ma-JŌra) extend down and back disappearing into the perineum behind. The labia majora contains sebaceous and sweat glands. Pubic hair grows on the outer part and the inner part is smooth.

Inside the labia majora are two smaller folds of skin called the labia minora (mī-NŌ-ra). They meet in front to form a hood-like structure called the prepuce (foreskin) that covers and protects the clitoris. The labia minora unite behind at the frenulum of the labia minora. The labia minora contain a number of sebaceous glands to lubricate the surface.

The clitoris (KLIT-o-ris) is a small sensitive organ containing erectile tissue and nerves. The exposed part of the clitoris is called the glans.

The cleft between the labia minora is called the vestibule and the orifice of the vagina and urethra open into it. The external urethral orifice lies at the back of the vestibule. At the entrance to the urethra there are two fine tubular glands called paraurethral or Skene's glands that secrete mucous. The orifice of the vagina is blocked by a crescent-shaped double fold of mucous membrane called the hymen. On either side of the vaginal orifice are two small glands, the greater vestibular or Bartholin's glands. The glands produce mucous during sexual arousal and intercourse.

The perineum (per'-iNĒ-um) is the diamond-shaped area of skin from the vaginal orifice back to the anus.

Vulva

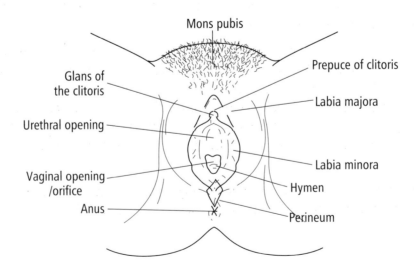

The internal female reproductive organs

Internal female reproductive organs

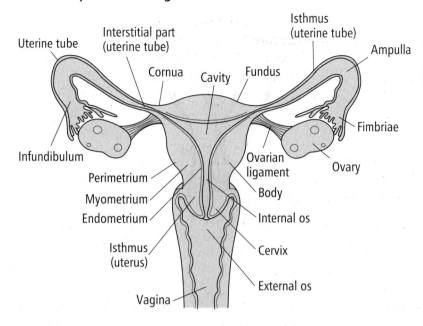

The vagina

The vagina (va-Jī-na) is a fibromuscular tube that creates a canal from the exterior skin to the uterus. It is situated between the urinary bladder and the rectum and it runs from the cervix to the vulva, at right angles to the axis of the uterus. The cervix enters the front wall of the vagina, making the back wall longer than the front.

A recess called the fornix surrounds the cervix, forming pockets called anterior, posterior and lateral fornices.

The wall of the vagina consists of fibrous and muscular tissue lined with mucous membrane. The mucous membrane of the vagina is continuous with that of the cervix and uterus. The lining is puckered with folds called rugae to allow for stretching during childbirth. The mucosa contains stores of glycogen. A by-product of the glycogen is organic acid which maintains an acidic environment that retards microbacterial growth and is harmful to sperm.

The smooth muscular layer allows the vagina to stretch to receive the penis during intercourse and to allow for menstrual flow and childbirth.

The uterus

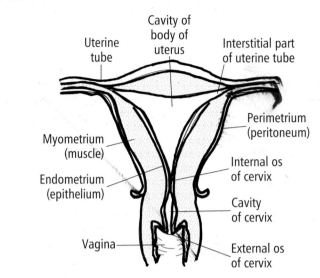

The uterus provides an environment in which to develop and nurture a growing fetus.

The uterus (womb) is a hollow, pear-shaped, muscular organ situated in the pelvic cavity between the urinary bladder and the rectum. The upper part is broad and dome-shaped and this portion is called the fundus. The mid-section is called the body and it contains a triangular cavity called the uterine cavity. Two fallopian tubes enter the uterus at the upper right angles of the cavity.

The body tapers downwards to the cervix. The cervix is a narrow opening with an internal and external os (os is an anatomical term for an opening). The cervix protrudes into the vagina.

The wall of the uterus consists of:

- Perimetrium: the outer covering.

- Myometrium: the middle layer of longitudinal, transverse and circular smooth muscle that produces coordinated contractions to help expel the fetus during childbirth.

- Endometrium: the inner lining of mucous membrane. There are two layers forming the endometrium:
    - Stratum basalis: the layer next to the myometrium.
    - Stratum functionalis (fungk'-shun-A-lis): this layer nourishes the growing fetus during pregnancy. If fertilisation of the ovum does not occur this layer is shed every 28 days or so during menstruation. Ovarian hormones promote regeneration.

The endometrium contains small tubular glands that secrete fluid to nourish sperm and the fertilised ovum (zygote).

The ovarian arteries and uterine arteries supply blood to the uterus. The arteries in the endometrium are adapted to degenerate with each menstrual flow.

The fallopian tubes

There are two fallopian tubes. Each one extends from the uterus into the peritoneal cavity. The tubes have a funnel-shaped end, the infundibulum, that divides into finger-like projections called fimbriae (FIM-brē-ē).

Section of the fallopian tube

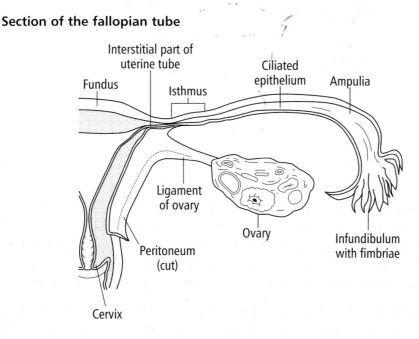

The fallopian tubes consist of:

- The infundibulum.

- The ampulla: the widest part of the tube.

- The isthmus: a narrow straight portion joining the ampulla to the uterus.

- The uterine or intramural part that lies within the wall of the uterus.

The tubes are made up of three layers of tissue:

- The outer layer: a serous membrane called the serosa.

- The middle layer – the muscularis: smooth muscle that contracts to provide a peristaltic action.

- The inner layer: a lining of ciliated epithelium containing secretory cells.

Function

The fallopian tubes convey the ovum from the ovary to the uterus. After ovulation the fimbriae move closer to the ovary causing the ovum to be swept up into the fallopian tube. The ovum is then moved along the tube by the ciliated epithelium and peristaltic action of the smooth muscle.

Fertilisation of the ovum by the sperm usually takes place in the fallopian tube.

The ovaries
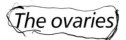

The ovaries are two small almond-shaped glands that produce secondary oöcytes (which become mature ova) and hormones including progesterone and oestrogen (female sex hormones).

They lie in the pelvic cavity, one either side of the uterus, and are held in place by the broad, ovarian and suspensory ligaments. Blood vessels, lymph and autonomic nerves enter the ovary at the hilum, which is the point of attachment for the broad ligament.

The ovaries consist of:

- The germinal epithelium: a layer of epithelium that covers the ovary.

- The cortex: the ovarian cortex is a layer of connective tissue called the stroma that contains ovarian follicles. Each follicle contains an oöcyte (sex cell).

In the fetus the ovaries and the sex cells (oöcytes) are developed by the fifth month. Many of these cells degenerate shortly before birth leaving approximately 40,000 oöcytes remaining at puberty. Of these, about 450 will mature and eventually be released at ovulation. The ovaries will release one mature ovum into the fallopian tube each month.

Puberty

In the ovary the oöcytes are surrounded by a layer of granulosa cells and this structure is called a primary follicle. Each month a group of follicles will begin a process in which the cells surrounding the oöcyte divide and grow, increasing the granulosa layers and producing a layer of glycoprotein.

The follicle now becomes known as a secondary follicle. The growth of follicles is stimulated by the follicule stimulating hormone (FSH) that is secreted by the pituitary gland.

As the cells continue to develop and mature, the surrounding cells secrete oestrogen. Oestrogen stimulates the endometrial lining of the uterus to grow. The secondary follicle develops an outer fibrous layer, a vascular layer and follicle fluid. The follicle matures and is called the graafian follicle.

Only one follicle is produced for ovulation, the others degenerate. Luteinising hormone (LH) secreted from the pituitary gland stimulates the process of ovulation. As blood levels of LH rise, the graafian follicle bursts open and releases the secondary oöcyte from the ovary (ovulation). The secondary oöcyte is swept into the fallopian tube.

Maturation of follicles

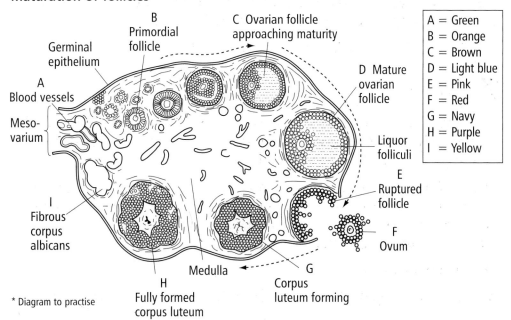

B
Primordial
follicle

C Ovarian follicle
approaching maturity

Germinal
epithelium

A
Blood vessels

Meso-
varium

I
Fibrous
corpus
albicans

D Mature
ovarian
follicle

Liquor
folliculi

E
Ruptured
follicle

F
Ovum

Medulla

G
Corpus
luteum forming

H
Fully formed
corpus luteum

* Diagram to practise

| A = Green |
| B = Orange |
| C = Brown |
| D = Light blue |
| E = Pink |
| F = Red |
| G = Navy |
| H = Purple |
| I = Yellow |

The area of the ovary where the graafian follicle has burst open fills with a blood clot and is then converted to a mass of cells known as the corpus luteum. If the secondary oöcyte is fertilised the corpus luteum remains and produces progesterone, oestrogens, relaxin and inhibin until the placenta is formed and takes over its function. If fertilisation does not take place the corpus luteum degenerates into fibrous tissue called a corpus albicans.

Egg

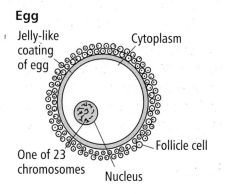

Jelly-like
coating
of egg

Cytoplasm

One of 23
chromosomes

Nucleus

Follicle cell

Fertilisation normally takes place in the fallopian tube. If sperm penetrates the secondary oöcyte, division will occur and an ovum or mature egg will be produced. If fertilisation does not occur the oöcyte passes into the uterus and is expelled during menstruation.

The menstrual cycle

The female reproductive cycle lasts for an average of 28 days. The menstrual cycle is divided into three phases:

- The menstrual phase: The first day of a new cycle starts on the first day of menstrual bleeding. This phase lasts for approximately 4–5 days. The discharge is due to the reduced levels of oestrogens and progesterone causing the uterus arteries to constrict. The stratum functionalis loses its blood supply and is expelled through the vagina. In the ovaries secondary follicles begin to enlarge.

- The pre-ovulatory or proliferative phase: The second phase begins when bleeding stops, and lasts for seven days. As the secondary follicles in the ovaries grow, oestrogen is produced. This stimulates the repair and growth of the endometrium in the uterus. Hormonal influences (including gonadatrophin-releasing hormone) prepare the mature graafial follicle to form a blister-like bulge on the surface of the ovary.

Ovarian and uterine cycles

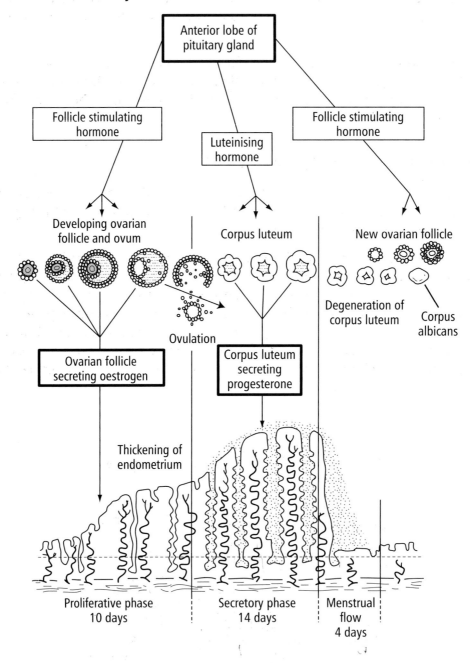

- Ovulation: The rupture of the graafial follicle and release of the secondary oöcyte occurs on day 14 of the menstrual cycle.

- The postovulatory or secretory phase: This phase lasts for approximately 14 days. Progesterone and oestrogen promote the growth of the endometrial glands and subsequent secretion of glycogen. The endometrium becomes thickened and vascular in preparation for the possible arrival of a fertilised ovum. If the oöcyte is not fertilised the decrease in progesterone and oestrogen gives rise to an increase in gonadotrophin-releasing hormone, follicle-stimulating hormone and luteinising hormone in order for a new cycle to begin.

If fertilisation has occurred, the corpus luteum continues to produce hormones as the embryo produces human chorionic gonadotrophin (hCG) hormone that stops it from degenerating. It is the presence of hCG in urine or blood that first indicates pregnancy.

Conception and fertilisation

Conception occurs when a spermatozoon reaches and penetrates a secondary oöcyte. Pregnancy is most likely to occur if sperm is introduced into the vagina two days before and one day after ovulation.

Of the 300–500 million sperm introduced into the vagina, only 100 will reach the vicinity of the oöcyte. This occurs within minutes of ejaculation. The sperm will undergo a change called capacitation which allows the release of enzymes necessary to fuse with the oöcyte's membrane. The first sperm to penetrate through the outer cover (the zona pellucida) fuses with the oöcyte. Within one to three seconds of fusion, chemical changes block fertilisation by other sperm. Once a sperm has fused with the oöcyte it divides into a mature egg called the

Conception

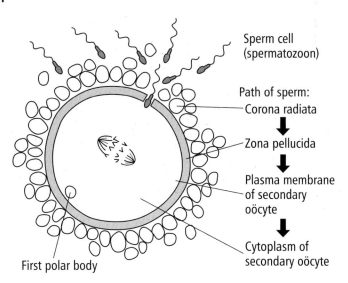

Sperm cell
(spermatozoon)

Path of sperm:
Corona radiata

Zona pellucida

Plasma membrane
of secondary
oöcyte

Cytoplasm of
secondary oöcyte

First polar body

ovum. Twenty-three maternal and 23 paternal chromosomes combine and the ovum is then fertilised and called a zygote (Zī-gōt).

The genetic sex of the baby depends on the sperm. The ovum carries the X chromosome and sperm may carry the X or Y chromosome. If the ovum is fertilised by sperm carrying the X chromosome it will produce a girl, if the sperm carries the Y chromosome it will produce a boy.

Determination of genetic sex

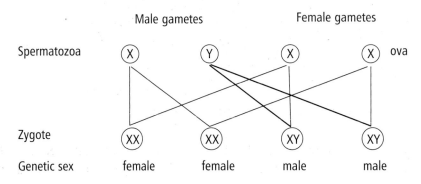

The zygote will begin to divide as it travels down through the fallopian tube to the uterus. The changes in the zygote produce a group of cells called the morula. The number of cells increase and after five days progress to the blastocyst stage. The blastocyst enters the uterus and after two days it will attach to the uterine wall, a process called implantation.

Fertilisation and implantation

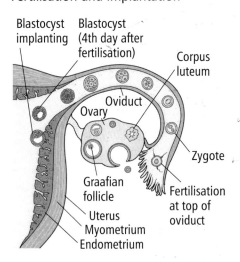

The placenta (pla-SEN-ta) develops between the inner mass of cells and the endometrium. The placenta will store nutrients and allow oxygen and nutrients to diffuse from maternal blood to fetal blood and transport waste products away from the fetus via the umbilical cord. It creates a barrier to microorganisms in order to protect the fetus. Certain viruses, alcohol and drugs will be able to cross the placenta barrier resulting in possible birth defects.

The fertilised embryo continues to develop, floating in a membrane filled with amniotic fluid which protects it. When the fetus fills the uterus, it will continue to grow and the uterus will expand and grow with it. Growth continues for 38 weeks, by which time the fetus will weigh, on average, 3.2 kg.

Placenta barrier

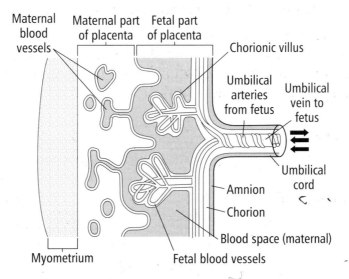

Maternal blood vessels — Maternal part of placenta — Fetal part of placenta — Chorionic villus — Umbilical arteries from fetus — Umbilical vein to fetus — Umbilical cord — Amnion — Chorion — Blood space (maternal) — Myometrium — Fetal blood vessels

The expected delivery date for the birth or parturition normally occurs 40 weeks from the first day of the last period. Labour is the common term used for childbirth and it occurs when the cervix dilates and the uterus contracts to expel the baby. After the birth of the baby the uterus contracts to separate the placenta and membranes from the uterine wall and expels them. The uterus will continue to contract in order to prevent excessive blood loss.

Stages of labour

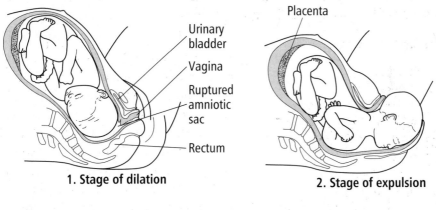

Urinary bladder — Vagina — Ruptured amniotic sac — Rectum

1. Stage of dilation

Placenta

2. Stage of expulsion

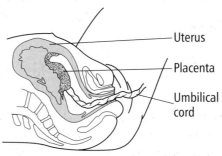

Uterus — Placenta — Umbilical cord

3. Placental stage

Following the birth the uterus and neighbouring structures will gradually return to their original size and position (this period is called the puerperium). This process, lasting six to eight weeks, is called involution and is due to self-digestion in the uterine cavity.

Lactation

Changes to the female breast occur during pregnancy and childbirth. The breasts are two glands responsible for lactation which includes the synthesis, secretion and ejection of milk. The breasts lie on the front aspect of the thorax and are attached to muscle by connective tissue. Each breast has a pigmented nipple which projects from the skin surface. The area around the nipple is called the areola and contains modified sebaceous glands. At the onset of puberty oestrogen and progesterone are produced that cause the glands to mature. Fat is deposited which increases breast size.

Mammary gland

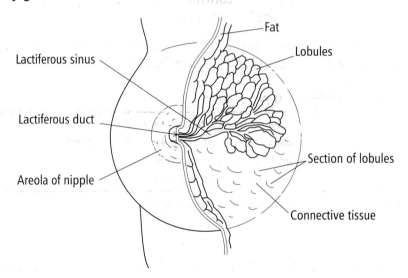

Mammary glands are modified sweat glands situated in the breast with the gland ducts converging into the nipple. The gland is divided into lobes that are subdivided into lobules. In each lobule are milk-secreting glands called alveoli.

Milk production is stimulated by the hormone prolactin. The ejection of the milk is the response to the act of breast-feeding the baby. When the baby is attached to the breast the pituitary gland releases oxytocin which promotes lactation.

Lactation

1. Prolactin secreted by anterior pituitary gland causes milk secretion by alveolar glands

2. Oxytocin released by posterior pituitary causes milk ejection as myoepithelial cells squeeze the glands and ducts

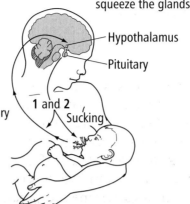

Hypothalamus

Pituitary

Impulses to hypothalamus and pituitary

1 and 2

Sucking

Hormones and pregnancy

The female reproductive cycle is controlled by gonadotrophin-releasing hormone (GnRH) secreted by the hypothalamus.

The physiological and psychological changes that occur during pregnancy are influenced by the secretion of hormones including the following.

Hormones produced during pregnancy

Progesterone	Essential to sustain the pregnancy Initiated by the corpus luteum and the placenta Inhibits uterine contractions Prepares breasts for lactation
Oestrogens	Produced by the corpus luteum Promotes growth of uterus Develops duct system of breasts Prepares uterine muscle for labour
Human chorionic gonadotrophin	Secreted by the developing ovum Maintains the corpus luteum secretion of hormones Presence in urine confirms pregnancy
Human placenta lactogen	Produced by the placenta Stimulates metabolism of carbohydrates and fat to produce glycogen for fetal use Prepares breasts for lactation
Oxytocin	Secreted by the posterior pituitary gland Initiates contractions for labour Contracts breast tissue to allow flow of milk during lactation Contracts uterus during involution of uterus
Relaxin	Produced by the placenta Increases flexibility of pelvic ligaments in preparation for labour

Menopause

The period of reproduction in women is limited to approximately 35 years. The menopause is the name given to the cessation of menstruation. The menopause occurs when the ovaries become less responsive to gonadatrophin hormones and the production of oestrogen falls. During this period ovulation becomes irregular and menstruation will eventually cease.

Birth control

Throughout the centuries different forms of birth control have been used in an attempt to prevent unintended pregnancy. Research to develop chemical contraceptives for men continues, but to date the responsibility for contraception remains predominately with women.

Biological, psychological and social influences will affect the method of birth control or contraception chosen. All methods used will have potential advantages and disadvantages.

Methods of birth control

Natural and mechanical methods	Advantages and disadvantages
Complete abstinence	100% reliable
Periodic abstinence (rhythm method): abstaining from sexual intercourse when signs of ovulation are present and for three days afterwards	The risk of pregnancy is reduced, but fertilisation is likely to occur if intercourse takes place up to two days before ovulation No protection from sexually transmitted diseases (STDs)
Coitus interruptus: removal of penis from the vagina before ejaculation	Very ineffective Pre-ejaculatory emission of sperm or failure to withdraw before ejaculation are the main reasons for the failure of this method No protection from STDs
Barrier methods 1(mechanical): condom and female condom	Prevents sperm entering the vagina. Effective if used correctly Provides protection against STDs
Diaphragm (cap): a dome-shaped rubber device that covers the entrance to the cervix	Used in conjunction with a spermicidal cream to kill the sperm it is very effective. No protection against STDs

Natural and mechanical methods	Advantages and disadvantages
Spermatocides in various forms including foams, creams, jellies and pessaries	Contain chemicals that kill sperm or make the vagina and cervix unsuitable for sperm survival High failure rate if used as the sole method of contraception but very effective if used in conjunction with a sheath or diaghragm No protection against STDs
Intrauterine device (IUD): a plastic device that is inserted into the uterus to prevent a fertilised ovum from implanting **An intrauterine device** One type of IUD Uterus 1 cm	An effective form of contraception, but IUDs are associated with pelvic inflammatory disease No protection against STDs

Hormonal methods of birth control	Advantages and disadvantages
Oral contraceptives: combined pills containing oestrogen and progesterone (includes 'morning after pill'). Promote low levels of FSH and LH to prevent follicular development and ovulation	Very effective if taken regularly. May cause high blood pressure in some women, smokers have an increased risk of heart attack or stroke Provides no protection from STDs
Progesterone only pill (mini pill). Promotes the formation of a mucous plug in the cervix to stop sperm entering	Effective if taken regularly at the same time each day Provides no protection from STDs
Norplant®. Six hormone-containing capsules are surgically inserted under the skin of the arm and they release progestin which inhibits ovulation and creates a mucus plug at the cervix. The capsules release the hormone for up to five years and may then be renewed	Very effective. Fertility is restored when capsules are removed. Offers no protection against STDs
Depo-provera®. An intramuscular injection given every three months. Contains progestin which prevents maturation of the ovum and stops changes in the lining of the uterus	Very effective Offers no protection against STDs

Surgical methods	Advantages and disadvantages
Removal of: • the testes (castration), or • the ovaries (oöphorectomy), or • the uterus (hysterectomy) An absolute and irreversible method that is not performed unless the organs are diseased	Removal of the testes or ovaries affects homeostasis due to the loss of endocrine secretions A hysterectomy will not affect the endocrine functions if the ovaries are left in situ Offers no protection against STDs
Vasectomy: male sterilisation Surgical procedure (usually under local anaesthetic) in which a portion of the vas deferens is removed so sperm can no longer be ejaculated. Spermatozoa remain in the epididymis and after vasectomy at least two checks are made to ensure the absence of sperm. The procedure may only be reversed by microsurgery **Vasectomy – both vas deferens are cut and tied** 	Very effective form of contraception Offers no protection against STDs

Surgical methods	Advantages and disadvantages
Tubal ligation: female sterilisation Surgical procedure (under general anaesthetic) in which the fallopian tubes are tied or clipped and then cut to prevent the secondary oöcyte and sperm meeting. The procedure may only be reversed by tubal microsurgery Tubal ligation: female sterilisation 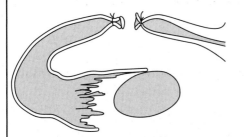	Very effective form of contraception Offers no protection against STDs
Induced abortion is a highly controversial form of contraception but may be deemed essential for the psychological and physical well-being of the woman. It involves removing the products of conception from the uterus. Induced abortion is usually performed in the first 12 weeks of pregnancy Certain drugs can induce the embryo to be aborted by blocking the action of progesterone. Drugs may be taken up to seven weeks after conception Anti-hCG vaccine may be used to inhibit the action of chorionic gonadotrophin and this will stimulate menstrual flow Surgical procedures: this may be achieved by vacuum aspiration (suction) or surgical evacuation (scraping) of the contents of the uterus	If surgical procedures are used there is a risk of damage to the cervix and uterus. Infection, haemorrhage and thrombosis are possible complications that may occur post-operatively. Induced abortion may have a detrimental effect on psychological health. The repeated use of induced abortions as a form of contraception increases the risk of psychological and physical damage to the woman No protection from STDs

4 Diseases and disorders of the reproductive system

Breast cancer

Breast cancer is caused by a change in the genetic composition of the cells. The abnormal cells divide rapidly and cause a mass of tissue called a tumour. The cells are capable of spreading to other sites in the body, causing secondary tumours to form. The most common sites for secondary tumours are the bone and liver.

Statstics show that the UK has the highest mortality rate in Europe for this disease and it is the most common form of cancer in women.

The cause of breast cancer is unknown. There is evidence to show that hereditary factors, gene BRA1, may increase the risk of the disease developing, but hormones and external environmental factors may also predispose the formation of cancer cells.

Treatment involves surgery, chemotherapy and/or radiotherapy, but the outcome will depend on the stage at which the disease was diagnosed. Early detection of a tumour by self-examination of breasts and yearly mammograms for women over the age of 50 are recommended in order to increase the chance of survival.

Cancer of the prostate gland

Prostate cancer is the third most common cancer in males and is treatable if detected in the early stages of development. There is an increased incidence with age, 80% of men over the age of 80 will have microscopic evidence of prostate cancer. The tumour/cancer cells are hormone dependent and usually grow very slowly. Blood tests to show levels of prostate-specific antigen may indicate infection, non-cancerous or cancerous tumours. Death from prostate cancer occurs due to metastases (spreading of cancer cells to other organs). Treatment is the surgical removal of the prostate gland, radiation, hormone treatment and/or chemotherapy.

Endometriosis (en'-dō-mē'-trē-Ō-sis)

In this condition the endometrium penetrates deep into the uterine wall causing the myometrium to thicken. Endometrial tissue may also be found outside the uterine wall on sites including the ovaries, sigmoid colon, abdominal wall and lymph nodes. Endometrial tissue responds to hormone control and the tissue will grow and then break down and bleed. This may cause pain and scarring to occur.

Sexually transmitted diseases

There are over 30 different types of virus, bacteria and parasites that cause sexually transmitted disease. Statistics gathered by the Public Health Laboratory Service at the Communicable Disease Surveillance Centre show that sexually transmitted disease affects over one million men and women in the UK each year.

The most recent STD to become identified is the human immunodeficiency virus (HIV) which causes acquired immune deficiency syndrome (AIDS). HIV can be transmitted during sexual contact, exchange of blood or through the placenta to the fetus.

Torsion of the testis

The spermatic cord containing the blood vessels for the testes may become twisted following physical exertion or trauma. It is common in young males and symptoms include severe pain, tenderness and swelling. Blood supply and venous drainage is compromised and unless the twist is reduced within six hours the testis will become necrotic (the tissue will die) leading to complete loss of function. This condition is treated as a surgical emergency and when the testis is untwisted it is anchored with a suture (stitch) to prevent reoccurrence. The unaffected testicle may also be anchored with a suture if there is an anatomical abnormality such as a long spermatic cord.

Sexually transmitted diseases

Disease	Cause	Symptoms
Chlamydia (kla-MID-ē-a)	Bacteria: Chlamydia trachomosis, transmitted through intimate physical contact. May be transferred on fingers from genitals to the eye and also from the mother to baby during birth	Females: 70% have no symptoms Increase of vaginal discharge due to inflammation of the cervix. Frequency and pain on passing urine Pain during sexual intercourse Pelvic inflammatory disease and infertility may result if condition remains untreated Males: Urethritis – frequent and painful urination

Disease	Cause	Symptoms
Genital herpes	Type2 herpes simplex virus	Produces painful blisters on the prepuce, glans penis, penile shaft, vulva or vagina. Blisters will disappear and reappear several times a year as the virus remains permanently in the body No cure available
Gonorrhoea (gon'-ōRĒ-a)	Bacteria: Neisseria gonorrhoeae, transmitted during sexual contact or mother to baby during birth	Females: Vaginal discharge. The bacteria spreads throughout the reproductive system and causes scar tissue leading to infertility. It is a cause of blindness in newborn babies delivered vaginally from an infected mother Males: Inflammation of the urethra (urethritis), painful urination and profuse pus discharge from urethra Treatable with antibiotics
Syphilis	Bacteria: Treponema pallidum, transmitted via sexual contact, exchange of blood or through the placenta to the fetus	There are three stages. **Primary:** a painless sore called a chancre appears and heals **Secondary:** infection spreads and becomes systemic – skin rash, fever, aches in muscles and joints. Then signs disappear. **Tertiary stage:** Organ degeneration occurs. Involvement of nervous system, including damage to the cerebral cortex, leads to neurosyphilis Treatable with antibiotics

Further reading

Aylin, P., Dunnell, K. and Drever, F. (1999) Trends in mortality of young adults aged 15–44 in England and Wales. *Health Statistics Quarterly*, Spring, 34–39.

Bailey, K. (2000) The nurse's role in promoting breast cancer. *Nursing Standard*, **14**(30), 34–36.

Harding, S., Brown, J., Rosato, M. and Hattersley, L. (1999) Socio-economic differentials in health: Illustrations from the Office for National Statistics Longitudinal Study. *Health Statistics Quarterly*, Spring, 8–10.

Zack, E. (2001) Mammography and reduced breast cancer mortality rates. *Medical Surgical Nursing*, **10**(1), 17–21.

Chapter 8

Defence systems

National unit specification
These are the topics you will be studying for this unit.

1   The lymphatic system

2   The immune system

3   Sensory organs

Diagrams to practise

Lymph node

Structure of the skin

Structure of the eye

Structure of the ear

Homeostasis

The lymphatic and immune system work together to defend the body against disease.

Skin:
Lymph vessels drain any excess interstitial fluid from the dermis.
The Langerhans cells help protect skin. Provides antibodies in sweat.
Eyelids and lashes protect vision.
Lacrimal secretions protect the eye surface by diluting microbes and washing them away.

Skeleton:
Drains excess interstitial fluid.

Muscular system:
Drains excess interstitial fluid.

Nervous system:
Drains excess interstitial fluid from the peripheral nervous system.
Memory and stress response act to avoid potential hazards using information from special senses from the peripheral nervous system.

Endocrine system:
Circulates and distributes hormones. Drains excess interstitial fluid.

Cardiovascular system:
Lymph returns fluid to the venous circulation.

Respiratory system:
Tonsils and mucous membranes act as a barrier to prevent entry of pathogens, thus protecting the lungs.
Cough reflex removes mucous and foreign bodies.
Drains excess interstitial fluid away.

Digestive system:
Antibodies present in saliva and digestive juices.
GI flora protects against pathogens.
Transports lipids and vitamins from the small intestines to the blood.
Drains excess interstitial fluid away.

Urinary system:
Lymph tissue helps to destroy pathogens in the urethra.
Urine flushes out pathogens in lower GU system.
Drains excess interstitial tissue away.

Reproductive system:
Lymph tissue defends against infections that gain entry via the vagina and penis.
Antibodies cross the placenta barrier to protect the fetus.
Antibodies present in human milk to increase immunity of feeding babies.
Drains excess interstitial fluid away.

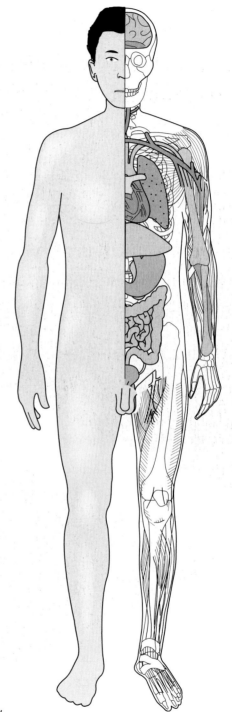

1 The lymphatic system

The lymphatic system is part of the body's defence system and a vital part of the cardiovascular system. Approximately 3 litres of interstitial fluid and proteins are returned to the cardiovascular system each day. Lymph fluid is similar to plasma except the solutions dissolved are in different concentrations.

Functions of the lymph system

- Draining interstitial fluid.

- Transporting cholesterol and vitamins A, D, E and K from the gastrointestinal tract to the blood.

- Protecting against foreign bodies, microbes and cancer cells.

Formation of lymph

Lymph is a clear watery fluid that consists of:

Water, Proteins, Fats, Hormones and Cellular waste.

Structures of the lymphatic system

Lymph capillaries

Capillaries begin as blind-ended tubes in tissue space. They have a single layer of endothelial cells. The capillaries join up to form lymph vessels.

Lymph capillaries collecting interstitial fluid

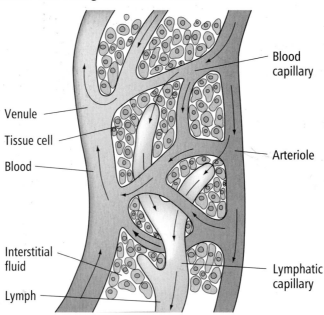

Venule

Tissue cell

Blood

Interstitial fluid

Lymph

Blood capillary

Arteriole

Lymphatic capillary

Lymph vessels

Lymph vessels are composed of three layers:

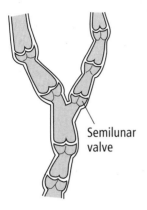

- Outer fibrous layer.

- Middle muscular, elastic layer.

- Inner layer of endothelial cells. The lining of the lymph vessels form semilunar valves to prevent backflow of lymph.

Semilunar valve

Lymph vessels transport lymph towards the heart and the flow of lymph depends on skeletal muscle movement and involuntary muscle movement during respiration.

Lymph ducts

The lymph is collected from the lymph vessels in the thoracic and right lymphatic duct. The thoracic duct receives lymph from the left side of the upper body and all of the lower body. The right lymphatic duct receives lymph from the right side of the upper body. The thoracic duct returns fluid to the cardiovascular system at a junction in the left jugular and subclavian vein. The right lymphatic duct returns fluid via a junction at the right jugular and subclavian vein.

Thoracic and right lymphatic duct

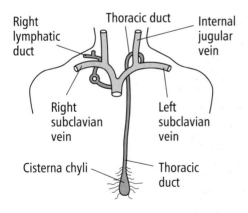

Right lymphatic duct

Thoracic duct

Internal jugular vein

Right subclavian vein

Left subclavian vein

Cisterna chyli

Thoracic duct

Areas drained by ducts

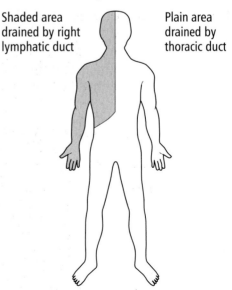

Shaded area drained by right lymphatic duct

Plain area drained by thoracic duct

Lymph nodes

Lymph nodes are situated throughout the lymphatic system and all lymph flow through at least one lymph node before returning to the blood. There are approximately 600 lymph nodes and they often occur in groups. Each node has a fibrous outer layer that also creates sections within the node called trabecule. Up to five lymph vessels (afferent vessels) may enter a lymph node, but only one or two will transport lymph away (efferent vessels). The lymph node acts as a filter, trapping foreign substances in the reticular fibres.

Lymph nodes contain lymphocytes, B cells that develop into plasma cells producing antibodies, and T cells that attack and destroy foreign cells and microbes. Macrophages are also present and they destroy pathogens by phagocytosis (fag'-ō-sī-TŌ-sis). Each node is covered with a capsule of fibrous tissue. The nodes contain lymphatic tissue.

A lymph node

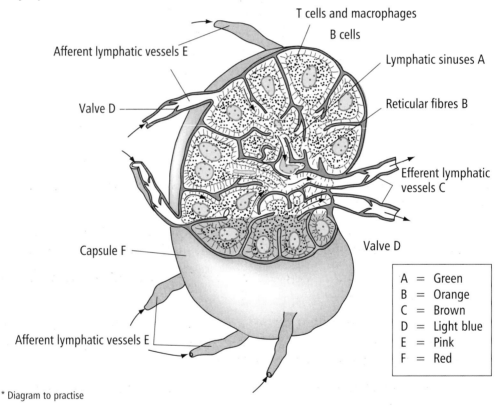

A	=	Green
B	=	Orange
C	=	Brown
D	=	Light blue
E	=	Pink
F	=	Red

* Diagram to practise

Lymphatic tissue

In addition to lymph nodes there are other sites containing lymphatic tissue. These sites include:

- The spleen.
- The tonsils.
- The thymus.

- Bone marrow.

- The liver.

- Peyer's patches in the small bowel.

- The appendix.

Location of lymph tissue

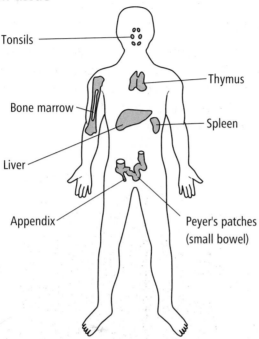

Tonsils

Thymus

Bone marrow

Spleen

Liver

Appendix

Peyer's patches
(small bowel)

The spleen is the largest body of lymphatic tissue, weighing approximately 200 g. The functions of the spleen include:

- Production of lymphocytes. T cells and B cells are produced which are capable of changing into cells that perform specific immune reactions.

- Phagocytosis: leucocytes, thrombocytes and microorganisms are phagocytosed in the spleen.

- Erythrocytes are destroyed in the spleen and the breakdown products bilirubin and iron are released from the haemoglobin and passed to the liver through the splenic and portal veins.

- Storage of platelets for use in emergency situations, for example hypoxia or severe haemorrhage.

Lymphatic circulation

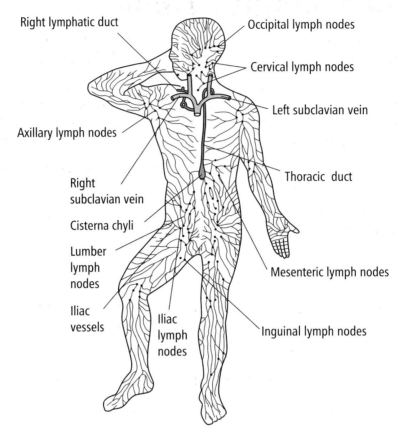

Right lymphatic duct

Occipital lymph nodes

Cervical lymph nodes

Left subclavian vein

Axillary lymph nodes

Thoracic duct

Right subclavian vein

Cisterna chyli

Lumber lymph nodes

Mesenteric lymph nodes

Iliac vessels

Iliac lymph nodes

Inguinal lymph nodes

2 The immune system

The human body is able to employ a wide variety of defences against disease-producing organisms (pathogens) in order to maintain homeostasis.

Resistance to disease is the ability to defend against certain pathogens by way of natural defences or immunity. Resistance to disease depends on many biopsychosocial factors. If conditions in the external environment are not conducive to health, susceptibility to disease may increase. The body has two areas of defence:

- Non-specific resistance: the body defends against pathogens by providing a rapid response to any invasion.

- Specific resistance: antibodies are produced to target specific pathogens thus producing immunity.

Natural defences

- Skin: prevents pathogens from entering the body by producing sebum, sweat and the process of shedding keratinised cells.

- Mucous membrane: produces mucous to trap pathogens.

- Hair and cilia: trap pathogens entering the respiratory tract.

- Saliva: flushes pathogens out of the oral cavity.

- Lacrimal glands: produce tears that contain the enzyme lysozyme to kill pathogens.

- Flow of urine: helps to wash out pathogens entering via the urethra.

- Acidic gastric environment: a pH of 1.3–3.0 in the stomach kills many pathogens. Vomiting expels pathogens.

- Vagina: secretions are slightly acidic.

- Brain: warns of danger by using memory and stress response.

If pathogens do enter the body a second line of defence systems come into action.

Antimicrobial proteins

Three main types of defence proteins are found in blood and lymph:

- Complement: when activated, the proteins are able to rupture the microbes, promote phagocytosis and cause inflammation.

- Transferrins: inhibit the growth of certain bacteria by reducing the amount of iron available.

- Interferon: stop viruses from replicating by producing antiviral proteins.

Phagocytes

Chemicals are released to attract phagocytes, a process called chemotaxis. Phagocytes, neutrophils and macrophages ingest microbes and debris. Lymphocytes contain natural killer cells that destroy microbes and tumour cells.

Inflammatory response

If cells are damaged they are protected and defended by a three-stage inflammatory response.

Inflammatory response

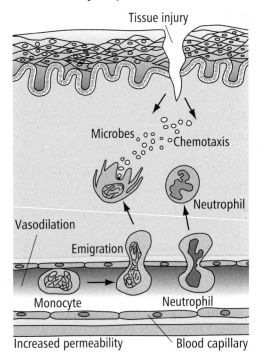

First stage

- Redness: vasodilation to increase blood flow.

- Pain: nerve endings damaged.

- Heat: due to increased blood flow to the damaged area.

- Swelling: increased interstitial fluid.

- Loss of function: depending on the severity of the damage.

Second stage

Emigration of phagocytes to ingest invading microbes.

Third stage

Repair of damage takes place. Pus is produced containing white blood cells and debris. If pus does not drain away from the site an abscess may form.

Immunity

When a foreign protein (antigen) enters the body the immediate response is the production of substances (antibodies) to react with it to render it harmless. This antigen–antibody reaction is called immunity. The human body is capable of producing millions of different types of antibodies. Antibodies remain in the blood to prevent further infection by the same type of virus or bacteria. In viruses such as the cold or flu virus there are many different strains, each with its own characteristic antigen, which means that colds and flu can reoccur.

Immunity may be active or passive.

Active immunity (when the body makes the antibody)

Active natural immunity

This is gained through contracting the disease or being exposed to small amounts of antigens that are insufficient to produce symptoms (called subclinical infections).

Active artificial immunity

This is gained by inoculation with living or dead viruses to stimulate the active natural immunity to develop antibodies.

- Dead virus: e.g. whooping cough.
- Live virus: made harmless by sub-culturing, e.g. rubella.
- Antigens: separated from the organism, e.g. influenza.
- Toxin: chemically modified poison, e.g. tetanus.
- Genetically engineered bacteria: for mass-produced antigen, e.g. hepatitis B.

Passive immunity (gained from another person)

Natural passive immunity

Antibodies are transferred from the mother to the fetus via the placenta, and mother to baby via breast milk. The antibodies are destroyed as the baby develops the ability to develop its own acquired immunity.

Artificial passive immunity

Innoculation of ready-made antibodies obtained from human or animal sera is administered prophylactically to prevent a person developing a disease if exposed to the pathogen. The serum (called anti-serum) is obtained from people who are convalescing from the disease or from horses that have been artificially immunised. Antibodies speed up the process of active immunity. The production of antibodies may take up to one week, but in cases of rabies and tetanus the introduction of antigens helps the body to fight the microorganisms immediately and thereby reduce the risk of fatality.

Abnormal immune responses

Allergies

The body's defence system is always alert to attack from harmful microorganisms. However, occasionally the immune system produces chemicals that

Immunity

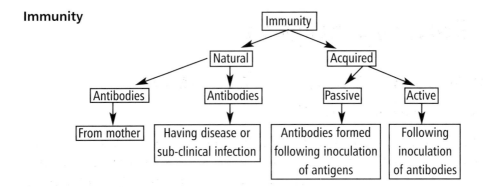

cause a hypersensitive reaction to an antigen resulting in an anaphylactic reaction or allergy.

An anaphylactic reaction may cause a variety of symptoms including skin redness (eczema), nasal discharge (hay fever) and bronchoconstriction (asthma). Reactions are usually more intense with each exposure to the antigen. In rare cases the reaction is so severe that a systemic reaction known as anaphylactic shock occurs. Following a second or repeated exposure to the antigen there is widespread release of chemicals that cause bronchospasm, oedema of the larynx and shock. The reaction is severe and requires immediate medical intervention. Bee stings, drugs (antibiotics) and peanut allergies are common causes of anaphylactic shock.

Autoimmune disorders

Body tissue contains different antigens that the immune system recognises and tolerates. Occasionally the tolerance mechanism fails spontaneously or due to drugs or disease. This results in the immune system destroying healthy tissue.

Immunodeficiency

Congenital or acquired defects of the immune system may result in the body being unable to produce sufficient antibodies to protect against harmful antigens. The body becomes susceptible to infection from all pathogens, including those that are normally viewed as harmless. Management of immunodeficiency includes isolating a person in a sterile environment to reduce the risk of infection.

Acquired immune deficiency syndrome (AIDS) develops following infection by the human immunodeficiency virus (HIV). The HIV infection attacks and fights cells of the immune system. This grossly impairs the immune system and normally harmless microbes can lead to fatal infections. When infection develops it signifies that the person has AIDS.

3 **Sensory organs**

The skin – the intergumentary system (in-teg'yoo-MEN-tar-ē)

The skin is the largest and most complex epithelial tissue in the body. It covers the whole body surface and lines the body orifices. Skin varies in thickness from half a centimetre on the soles of the feet to approximately half a millimetre on the eyelids.

Functions of the skin

- Protection against:
  - Potential pathological organisms.
  - Chemical damage.
  - Physical injury.
  - Ultraviolet radiation from the sun.
  - Dehydration.
- Temperature control:
  - Sweating.
  - Changes in blood flow to the skin.
  - Movement of hair.
- Sensory:
  - Contains receptors for touch, pain, pressure and temperature.
- Excretion and secretion:
  - Water and salts are excreted by sweat glands.
  - Oils secreted by sebaceous glands keep the skin supple.
- Immunity:
  - Contains cells designed to defend against harmful microbes.
- Vitamin D production:
  - Ultraviolet rays are absorbed which are needed to begin production of vitamin D.

Changes in skin, such as colour, integrity, heat, swelling or pain may indicate homeostatic imbalances due to systemic or localised disease and disorders.

As skin is the most visible component of our body it also helps to express our emotions and body image. Becoming 'red with embarrassment' or 'pale with fright' indicates our emotional state. Skin degenerates with age, prompting many people to explore ways of retaining or restoring a youthful complexion in order to maintain their body image.

Health and appearance of skin is affected by many factors including diet, hygiene, circulation, age, external environmental factors (sun, wind, pollution etc.), mobility and psychological health.

Structure of the skin

Skin is composed of two layers: the outer, thinner layer of epidermis (ep'-I-DERM-is) and the thicker dermis with a deep layer of hypodermis (subcutaneous tissue).

Section through the skin

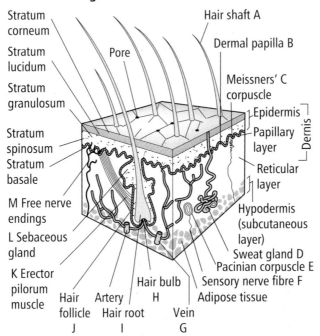

Stratum corneum
Stratum lucidum
Stratum granulosum
Stratum spinosum
Stratum basale
M Free nerve endings
L Sebaceous gland
K Erector pilorum muscle
Hair follicle J
Artery
Hair root I
Hair bulb H
Vein G
Pore
Hair shaft A
Dermal papilla B
Meissners' C corpuscle
Epidermis
Papillary layer
Dermis
Reticular layer
Hypodermis (subcutaneous layer)
Sweat gland D
Pacinian corpuscle E
Sensory nerve fibre F
Adipose tissue

A	=	Brown
B	=	Green
C	=	Orange
D	=	Light Blue
E	=	Pink
F	=	Red
G	=	Dark blue
H	=	Yellow
I	=	Purple
J	=	Light green
K	=	Lilac
L	=	Tan
M	=	Dark orange

* Diagram to practise

Epidermis

The epidermis is composed of multiple layers of stratified squamous epithelia. The thickness of the layers depends on the amount of friction it is exposed to. The epidermis consists of five layers:

- Stratum corneum (COR-ne-um): horny layer shedding dead skin cells, a process called desquamation.

- Stratum lucidum (LOO-si-dum): clear layer.

- Stratum granulosum (gran-yoo-LŌ-sum): granular layer.

- Stratum spinosum (spi-NŌ-sum): prickle cell layer.

Layers of the epidermis

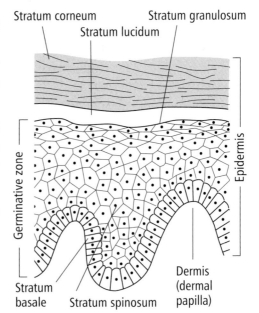

Stratum corneum
Stratum granulosum
Stratum lucidum
Epidermis
Germinative zone
Stratum basale
Stratum spinosum
Dermis (dermal papilla)

The cells of the basal layer (furthest from the surface of the skin) of the epidermis are constantly dividing and as they move towards the surface they become flatter in shape. As they reach the surface they make keratin, a protein that protects skin from heat and microbes and helps to make it waterproof. The keratinised top layer is lost by normal abrasion and is replaced by the cells below. The epidermis has no blood supply and little nerve supply. It is nourished by lymph from underlying vessels.

The basal layer contains melanocytes (MEL-a-nō-sīts) that produce the pigment melanin which gives skin its colouration. Melanin production is activated by ultraviolet light.

Langerhans (LANG-er-hans) cells migrate to the epidermis from red bone marrow. These cells help to protect the skin from microbes.

Merkel cells located in the basal layer produce the sensation of touch as they press on sensory nerves in the dermis.

The dermis

The dermis is a tough, thick layer of connective tissue containing collagen and elastin fibres, and it lies beneath the epidermis. This layer provides the skin with its strength and elasticity. The uppermost surface of the dermis has small projections called dermal papillae (pa-PIL-ē) that contain touch-sensitive receptors called Meissner's corpuscles and blood vessels. The dermal papillae cause ridges in the epidermis and this is seen on the fingers as fingerprints.

Meissner's corpuscle

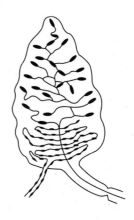

A hair follicle

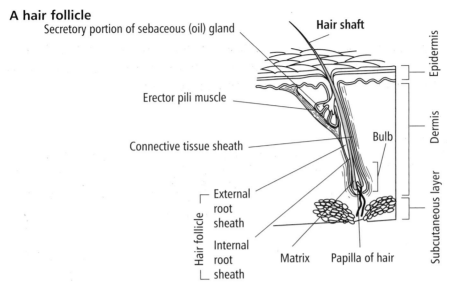

The deeper layers of the dermis contain:

- Sebaceous glands: that secrete sebum into hair follicles to keep hair soft. On the skin sebum acts as a bactericidal agent, it provides a waterproofing effect and prevents skin drying out in heat.

Sweat gland

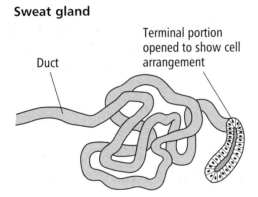

- Hair follicles: a downward growth of epidermal cells. At the bottom of each follicle is a cluster of cells called the bulb. The cells multiply to form the hair. The hair seen on the body is keratinised (dead cells). The erector pili muscles are attached to hair follicles. They contract and move the hair in response to cold or fear.

- Sudiferous (sweat) glands: there are two types of sweat glands both composed of epithelial cells. Eccrine glands are found in most areas of skin and are responsible for the excretion of water, urea, salt ions and toxins. Apocrine glands open into the hair follicles of the armpit, axilla/pubic area and areola of the breasts. The most important function of sweat is to assist in regulation of body temperature.

- Nerves: sensory nerve endings relay messages to the hypothalamus. The skin is an important sensory organ as it allows the body to be aware of the external environment.

Subcutaneous layer

This layer attaches the dermis to underlying bone and muscle. It consists mainly of fat and it functions as an insulating layer to help maintain body temperature and also as an energy store. The thickness of this layer varies greatly between individuals and differs depending on the area of the body that it is covering.

Nails

Nails are hard keratinised plates of modified epithelium that protects the tips of the digits (fingers and toes). Nail growth occurs in the nail matrix. Nails assist in the function of grasping and manipulating small objects.

Structure of a fingernail

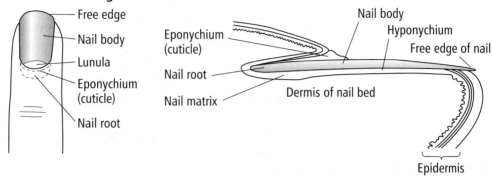

Skin conditions

Acne vulgaris

Acne is caused by an inflammation of the sebaceous glands due to bacterial infection. It is a common condition during puberty and if severe may result in the formation of scar tissue. Treatments are localised (i.e. lotions/creams) or long-term systemic antibiotics.

Eczema

Eczema is an inflammatory response to chemical agents. The cause may be a reaction to substances in the sebum or a dermatitis caused by allergy or an irritant.

Malignant melanoma

This is the most common type of skin cancer often resulting from over-exposure to ultraviolet rays from the sun or tanning equipment. Melanoma is a cancer of the pigmented melanocytes and unless diagnosed and treated in the early stages it will invade surrounding tissue and send metastases (malignant cells) to lymph nodes, the liver, lungs, bone and the brain. The use of wide-brim hats, sun block and limited exposure to harsh ultraviolet light is recommended to reduce the incidence of melanomas.

Warts

Warts are caused by a virus called papovavirus. Cells react by dividing excessively to produce a small raised area of hard skin. If the virus enters the soles of the feet the hard skin is pushed inwards due to the pressure/weight of the body, creating a verucca.

The eye

The eye is the organ of sight and it is situated in the orbital cavity. Vision requires detection of light and colour.

The eye and accessory structures

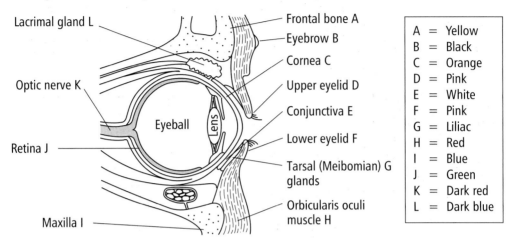

Lacrimal gland L
Optic nerve K
Retina J
Maxilla I
Eyeball
Lens

Frontal bone A
Eyebrow B
Cornea C
Upper eyelid D
Conjunctiva E
Lower eyelid F
Tarsal (Meibomian) G glands
Orbicularis oculi muscle H

A	=	Yellow
B	=	Black
C	=	Orange
D	=	Pink
E	=	White
F	=	Pink
G	=	Liliac
H	=	Red
I	=	Blue
J	=	Green
K	=	Dark red
L	=	Dark blue

Light rays are reflected from an object to the cornea. The rays are bent and focused by the cornea, lens and vitreous fluid to provide a clear upside-down image on the retina. The light rays are converted to electrical impulses and sent via the optic nerve to the brain. The eye contains over half of the sensory receptors in the body, so the sense of sight can supply the brain with a vast array of information about the external environment. The muscles of both eyes work in unison to allow the eyes to work in coordination with each other. It is possible to see with one eye but three-dimensional vision will be impaired (making it difficult to judge the distance of an object).

The orbit of the eye is a conical-shaped depression made up of several different skull bones. Six extraocular muscles are attached to the wall of the eye to allow coordinated movement.

Muscles that control eye movement

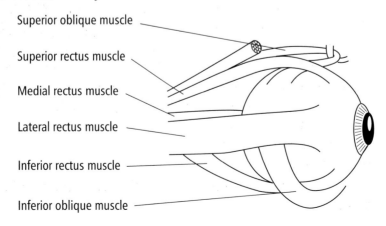

Superior oblique muscle
Superior rectus muscle
Medial rectus muscle
Lateral rectus muscle
Inferior rectus muscle
Inferior oblique muscle

Structure

Cross-section of the eye

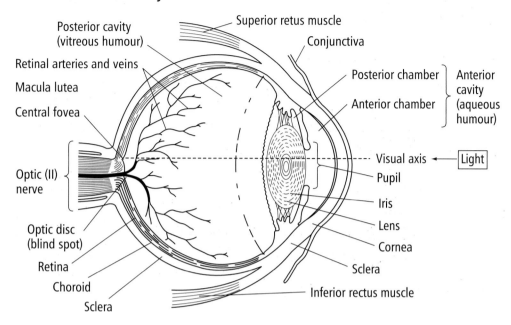

The wall of the eye has three layers:

- Sclera (SKLER-a): an outer layer of tough white connective tissue that gives shape and strength to the eye. At the front of the eye it becomes a non-vascular transparent layer called the cornea (KOR-nē-a). The cornea bends light.

- Choroid (KOR-oyd): a thin vascular layer that nourishes the retina and lines five-sixths of the inner surface of the sclera.

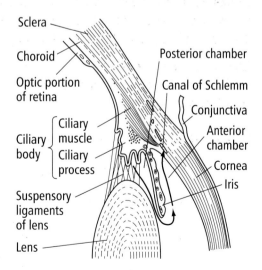

At the front of the eye the choroid forms a ring-shaped structure called the ciliary body (SIL-ē-ar′-ē). The ciliary body consists of ciliary muscle and epithelial tissue. It provides attachment to the suspensory ligament that holds the lens in place.

Contraction and relaxation of the ciliary muscle changes the thickness of the lens. The lens refracts (bends) the light rays entering the eye to focus them on the retina.

The epithelial tissue secretes aqueous fluid into the space in front of the lens (anterior segment).

The iris is the coloured portion of the eye containing pigment to prevent light passing through, and it is situated in front of the lens. The iris contains circular and longitudinal smooth muscle that is attached to the front of the ciliary body.

In the centre of the iris is an aperture (hole) known as the pupil.

Pupils reacting to light

Dim light   Bright light

1 Circular muscle relaxed
2 Radial muscle contracted
Pupil dilated (large)

1 Circular muscle contracted
2 Radial muscle relaxed
Pupil constricted (small)

Light passes through the pupil to the back of the eye. The strength of the light will alter the size of the pupil. In bright light the circular muscle contracts and the pupil constricts (becomes smaller), and in dim light the longitudinal muscle contracts and the pupil dilates (becomes larger).

The two pupils are normally equal in size and are innervated by the autonomic nervous system.

- Retina: the retina forms the inner layer of the eye. The retina contains highly specialised cells called photoreceptors that convert light impulses to electrical charges which are conducted via nerve cells to the optic nerve at the back of the orbit.

Optic nerves and the optic tract

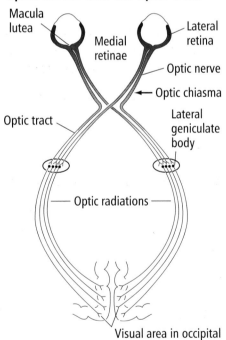

Macula lutea

Medial retinae

Lateral retina

Optic nerve

Optic chiasma

Lateral geniculate body

Optic tract

Optic radiations

Visual area in occipital lobe of cerebrum

Photoreceptors are the sensory and receptor nerve endings, often called rods and cones. The rods are light sensitive for vision in dim light and the cones are responsible for colour vision.

Cones are concentrated in one area of the retina called the fovea. There are no receptors at the point where the optic nerve leaves the eye and this is called a blind spot.

Nerve impulses pass to the thalamus and are then relayed to the occipital cortex.

The inner globe of the eye is filled with a clear jelly-like substance called the vitreous body. It provides support and pressure to maintain the shape of the eye.

Rods and cones

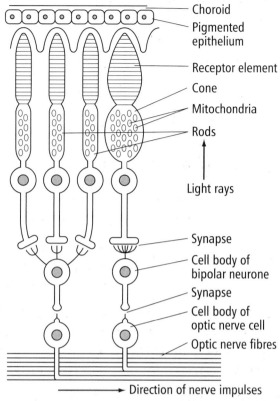

The labels in the diagram:
- Choroid
- Pigmented epithelium
- Receptor element
- Cone
- Mitochondria
- Rods
- Light rays
- Synapse
- Cell body of bipolar neurone
- Synapse
- Cell body of optic nerve cell
- Optic nerve fibres
- Direction of nerve impulses

The conjunctiva

The conjunctiva is a thin vascular membrane that covers the internal surfaces of the eyelids and the visible portion of the sclera. If the conjunctiva is touched, even very lightly or as a response to fear of injury, the eyelids will automatically close.

When the eyelids are closed the conjunctiva forms a sac-like structure to protect the front of the eye and the cornea.

The lacrimal apparatus

The lacrimal apparatus consists of the glands, ducts, canals and sacs that secrete and drain tears.

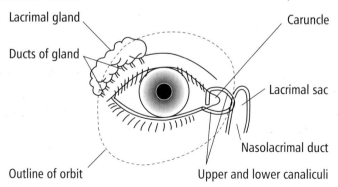

Labels in the diagram:
- Lacrimal gland
- Ducts of gland
- Caruncle
- Lacrimal sac
- Nasolacrimal duct
- Upper and lower canaliculi
- Outline of orbit

Tears consist of water, salts and lysozyme – a bactericidal protein. Tears are constantly produced to moisten and clean the outer surface of the eye. Drainage of tears takes place via the nasolacrimal duct.

In emotional states parasympathetic stimulation may produce tears that over-flow the edges of the eyelids.

Diseases and disorders of the eye

Cataracts

A cataract is a lens that has lost its transparency and has become cloudy or opaque. This prevents light from entering the eye, resulting in blindness. Age-related degenerative changes are a frequent cause of cataracts in older people. Cataracts may also be congenital (babies are sometimes born with cataracts), due to systemic diseases (e.g. diabetes), side effects of drugs (e.g. corticos-teroids) or as a result of trauma. Treatment consists of removing the lens and implanting an artificial lens or wearing spectacles with special lenses.

Corneal abrasion

The surface of the cornea is very sensitive. If a foreign body, dust, sand particles, metal splinters etc. scratch the cornea the pain is severe and it is accompanied by excessive tear production. A scratch usually heals after a period of 24 hours. Occasionally the cornea may be left with scar tissue after healing has taken place. Scar tissue is not transparent and will therefore affect sight to some degree. Exposure to very bright light or prolonged ultraviolet light may cause corneal burns. The burns are very painful but usually heal without scarring.

Damaged cornea may be removed and then replaced with donor corneas. As the cornea has no blood supply the risk of rejection of the tissue implant is greatly reduced.

The ears

The ear is the organ for hearing and it allows us to respond to and enjoy a wide range of sounds and helps to maintain balance.

Parts of the ear

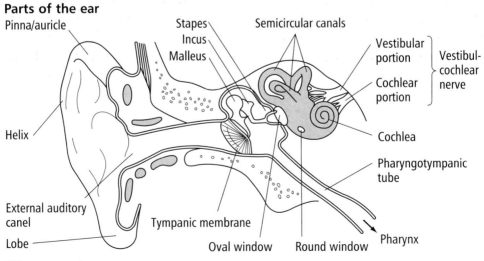

* Diagram to practise

Structure

The ear is made up three of three distinct parts.

The external ear

The auricle (or pinna) is the part of the ear that is attached to the side of the head. It is composed of fibroelastic cartilage and is covered with skin. Its function is to collect sound waves and conduct them to the external auditory meatus.

The external auditory meatus is a canal (tube) that leads from the auricle to the tympanic membrane (ear drum). Cartilaginous tissue lines one-third of the canal and contains modified sweat glands called ceruminous glands (se-ROO-mi-nus) that secrete ear wax called cerumen (se-ROO-min). The wax helps to protect the inner ear by trapping dust or other foreign material.

The tympanic membrane (tim-PAN-ik) separates the external auditory meatus from the middle ear.

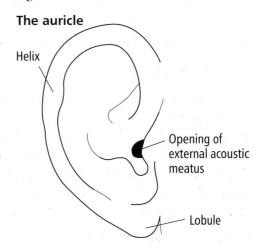

The auricle

Helix

Opening of external acoustic meatus

Lobule

The tympanic cavity

The tympanic cavity is an irregular-shaped air-filled cavity. The air pressure in the cavity is the same as atmospheric pressure. The air comes from a tube called the eustachian tube that links the ear with the nasopharynx. Air pressure on both sides of the tympanic membrane allows it to vibrate with sound waves.

The tympanic cavity contains a chain of three minute bones – the malleus, incus and stapes (commonly called the hammer, anvil and stirrup) – known as the auditory ossicles. The bones extend across the cavity and form a series of movable joints. Sound waves are transmitted from the tympanic membrane through the auditory ossicles to the fenestra ovalis, an oval window of membrane connecting with the internal ear.

The tympanic cavity and inner ear

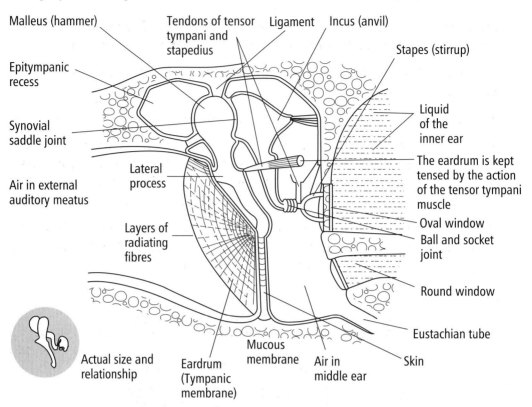

Malleus (hammer)

Tendons of tensor tympani and stapedius

Ligament

Incus (anvil)

Stapes (stirrup)

Epitympanic recess

Synovial saddle joint

Air in external auditory meatus

Lateral process

Layers of radiating fibres

Liquid of the inner ear

The eardrum is kept tensed by the action of the tensor tympani muscle

Oval window

Ball and socket joint

Round window

Eustachian tube

Actual size and relationship

Eardrum (Tympanic membrane)

Mucous membrane

Air in middle ear

Skin

The auditory ossicles

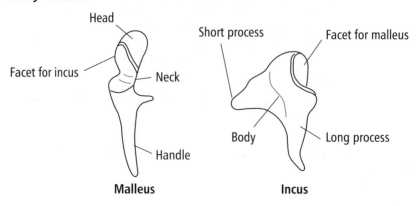

Head

Facet for incus

Neck

Handle

Malleus

Short process

Facet for malleus

Body

Long process

Incus

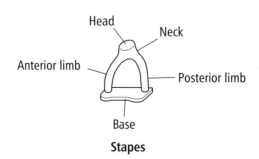

Head

Neck

Anterior limb

Posterior limb

Base

Stapes

The internal ear

The internal ear (labyrinth) contains the bony labyrinth of cavities that enclose a similar-shaped membrane structure called the membranous labyrinth.

Perilymph fluid separates the walls of the bony and membranous labyrinths. The bony labyrinth is divided into three parts:

- One vestibule: the vestibule is the expanded area nearest to the middle ear.

- One cochlea: the cochlea is shaped like a snail shell. The cochlea contains auditory receptors that transmit messages to the brain via the organ of corti and auditory nerve. It receives information from the perilymph fluid that transmits vibrations from the fenestra ovalis to the cochlea.

- Three semicircular canals: the semicircular canals are a continuation of the vestibule and they contain receptors that are concerned with equilibrium (balance); they have no auditory (hearing) function.

Organ of corti

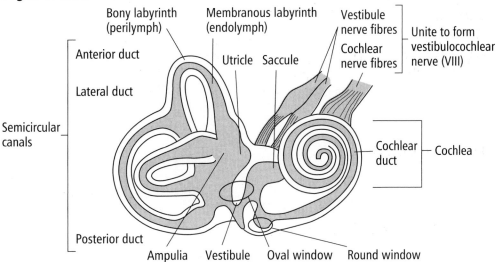

For hearing to be achieved, sound waves must pass through the following:

- The pinna.
- External canal.
- Tympanic membrane.
- Ossicles.
- Oval window.
- Perilymph.
- Endolymph.
- Organ of corti to the auditory nerve pathway.

Auditory nerve pathway

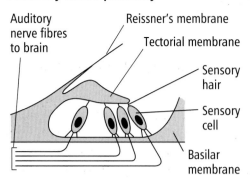

Auditory nerve fibres to brain

Reissner's membrane

Tectorial membrane

Sensory hair

Sensory cell

Basilar membrane

Receptor for balance

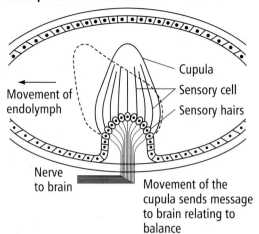

Cupula

Sensory cell

Sensory hairs

Movement of endolymph

Nerve to brain

Movement of the cupula sends message to brain relating to balance

Hearing pathway

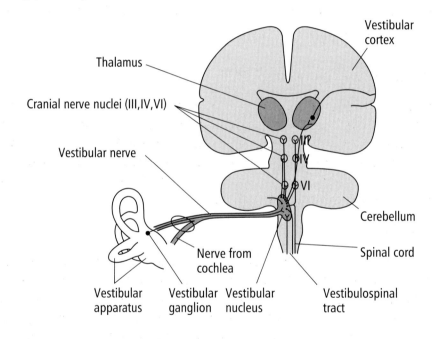

Vestibular cortex

Thalamus

Cranial nerve nuclei (III, IV, VI)

Vestibular nerve

III

IV

VI

Cerebellum

Spinal cord

Nerve from cochlea

Vestibulospinal tract

Vestibular apparatus

Vestibular ganglion

Vestibular nucleus

Disease and disorders of the ear

Deafness

Deafness is the partial or complete loss of hearing in one or both ears. There are two types of deafness:

- Conductive deafness: caused by faulty external and middle ear transmissions of sound. A common cause of conductive deafness in adults is ear-wax. Otosclerosis is a condition in which deposits of new bone are placed around the oval window and if deafness occurs surgery to replace the stapes is required.

- Sensorineural deafness: in which there is a failure in transmission of sounds to the brain. The hair cells in the cochlea or nerve are damaged at birth or later in life. Noise pollution, viral infection, artherosclerosis or drugs such as aspirin may cause sensorineural damage.

During the ageing process deafness occurs due to natural degeneration of the cochlea and labyrinth.

Menière's disease

Menière's disease is an inner ear disorder that is brought about by an increase of endolymph fluid in the labyrinth which causes a syndrome of vertigo (feeling of spinning), tinnitus (ringing noise) and deafness. Symptoms may last for minutes or hours and may be accompanied by nausea and vomiting and hearing loss. Drugs or surgery are necessary to control the symptoms. Total loss of hearing may occur after a period of time.

Otitis media

The eustachian tube may allow bacteria from the nasopharynx to enter the middle ear. This causes inflammation called otitis media. It is common in young children and they complain of earache usually accompanied by a raised temperature. Treatment with antibiotics is usually required to prevent progress of the infection. The inflammation may be accompanied with the formation of pus, reducing hearing ability by increasing the pressure in the middle ear, commonly called glue ear.

Smell and taste

The senses of smell and taste also send messages to the brain concerning the external environment. The diagrams below show the structure of the organs responsible for relaying messages of smell and taste.

Smell – olfaction

The receptors for smell are in the olfactory epithelium in the upper part of the nose. Each odour is made up of molecules and the molecules are dissolved in mucous before information is passed on to the olfactory receptors. There are between 10 and 100 million receptors in the nose and we are able to recognise approximately 10,000 different scents.

Olfactory structure

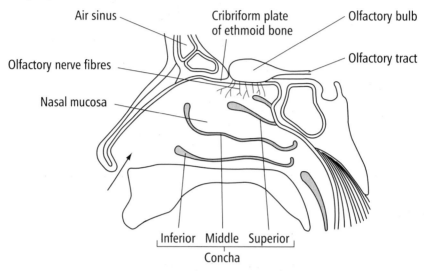

Olfactory receptors

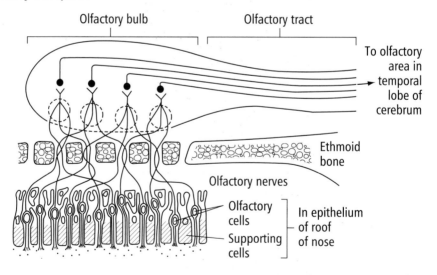

Taste – gustation

The receptors for taste are located in the taste buds on the tongue. Substances are dissolved in saliva before the receptors can distinguish the four primary tastes of bitter, sweet, sour and salty.

Tongue

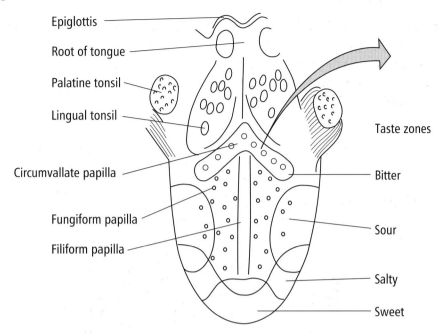

Epiglottis
Root of tongue
Palatine tonsil
Lingual tonsil
Circumvallate papilla
Fungiform papilla
Filiform papilla

Taste zones
Bitter
Sour
Salty
Sweet

Taste buds

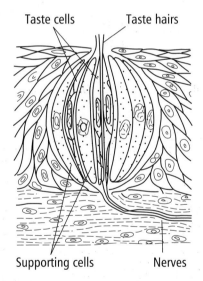

Taste cells   Taste hairs

Supporting cells   Nerves

Gustatory pathway

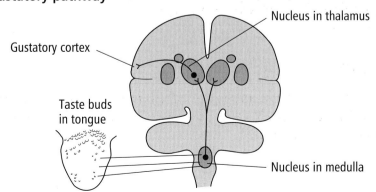

Nucleus in thalamus
Gustatory cortex
Taste buds
in tongue
Nucleus in medulla

Further reading

Arnould-Taylor, W. (2001) *A Textbook of Anatomy and Physiology*, 3rd edn. Nelson Thornes Ltd, Cheltenham.

Clancy, J. and McVicar, A. (2002) *Physiology and Anatomy: A Homeostatic Approach*, 2nd edn. Arnold, London.

Fullick, A. (2000) *Biology*. Heinemann, Oxford.

Muke, B., Inge, B. and Senior, K. (1999) *Understanding Advanced Human Biology*. HarperCollins, London.

Thompson, H. and Manuel, J. (2000) *Further Studies for Health*. Hodder and Stoughton, London.

Tortora, G. and Grabowski, S. (2001) *Introduction to the Human Body*, 5th edn. Wiley & Sons, New York.

Vellacott, J. and Side, S. (1999) *Understanding Advanced Human Biology*. Hodder and Stoughton, London.

Chapter 9
Stress and illness

National unit specification
These are the topics you will be studying for this unit.

1 Defining stress

2 Identifying stressors

3 Signs and symptoms of stress

4 Physiological responses to stress

5 Models of stress

6 Measuring stress

7 How stress affects health

8 Coping mechanisms, responses and strategies

9 Techniques to improve coping strategies

10 Controlling physiological effects of stress

Homeostasis

Stress is identified by a disturbed homeostastis that affects all systems within the body:

Skin:
Vasoconstriction. Cold hands and feet. Sweaty palms.

Cardio vascular:
Increased cardiac output heart rate.
Blood pressure.

Respiratory:
Respiratory rate.
Dilation of bronchus.

Urinary system:
Production of urine to maintain circulatory fluid volume.
Sensation for frequency of micturition.

Reproductive system:
Sexual libido decreases and causes ammenhoria.
Sexual dysfunction.

Muscles:
Dilation of arterioles supplying skeletal muscle,
cardiac muscle.

Nervous system:
Increased arousal. Pain threshold increased.

Gastrointestinal:
Constriction of arterioles.
Mobility.
Constipation or diarrhoea.
Gastric acid.
Nausea.

Skeletal system:
Back pain.

Endocrine:
Catecholmines.
ACTH.
Corlicosteroid.

Lymphatic system:
Decrease mass of lymph tissue.
WBC production and circulating lymphocytes.

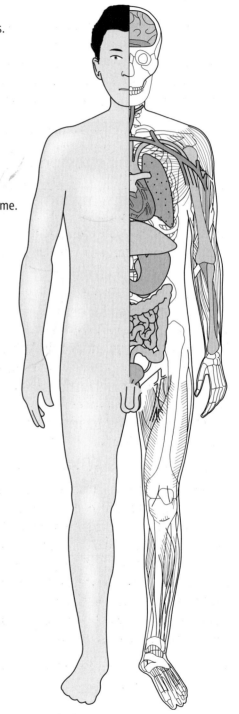

1 Defining stress

Stress

Unbelievable as it may sound, we all need stress in our lives. Stress motivates us to complete basic daily tasks and to aim higher to achieve personal goals. The feeling of stress and our stress response is a complex mixture of thought processes, physiological changes and behaviour patterns. The experience of stress is caused by stimuli (called stressors) that the body must adapt to.

To investigate how stress relates to illness it is necessary to define stress and identify the signs and symptoms of stress. The effect of stress on our well-being is investigated using different models and theories that identify physical and psychological effects on the human body.

Coping mechanisms allow different personalities to respond in different ways to stressors and the effects of stress. How a person copes with stress will depend on physiological, psychological and social factors.

Stress and illness

The early Greek philosophers believed that the mind (thoughts and feelings) and the body were separate and did not directly influence one another, and this philosophy continued throughout the centuries. In the nineteenth century the biomedical model of disease was established which explained illness solely in terms of biological processes. In industrialised countries this model has helped to establish many cures for disease, but it fails to fully describe the cause and prevention of illness.

In the mid twentieth century it was recognised that the study of illness required more than just the knowledge of anatomy and physiology. Knowledge of other factors that relate to health helped to establish a far greater understanding of how illness was linked to a person's internal and external environment. The biopsychosocial model of health (Engel, 1980) provides a framework of care that takes into account all of the processes involved in the study of health and illness. By studying the relationship between biological, psychological and social factors, healthcare workers are able to provide holistic care for clients rather than just treating the biological cause of an illness. This model of health allows the health-care worker to examine health and illness by exploring different areas including:

- The macro-level: main factors of health and illness including treatment or support available.

- The micro-level: minute causes, including chemical imbalance, that affect health.

- Multi-causal factors: different factors that work together to affect health and illness.

- Psychophysical: the relationship between mind and body and how they work together during health and illness.

The relationship between stress and illness illustrates the link between physiology, psychology and sociological factors creating a multi-causal situation that may have an adverse effect upon health.

What is stress?

As an Access student you may have already experienced stress, and you will understand if fellow students say that they are feeling stressed. The word 'stress' may be used in a positive or negative way and in general the word is used to indicate some form of demand being made and your ability to cope with that demand.

Stress is a frequently used word and has a variety of distinctive meanings when used by different groups of people, i.e. engineers, psychologists, business and healthcare professionals, and therefore it is quite difficult to give an overall definition.

For those studying healthcare, stress may be defined as a state of potential challenge or threat that is perceived as presenting a demand that exceeds the adaptive capacities of an individual's mind and body. The term 'stress' therefore refers to an imbalance between the demands of a situation, called a stressor, and an individual's physical or psychological ability to cope.

Potential demands, threats or challenges are essential in everyday life as they help us to perform routine tasks. In this respect stress is viewed as positive as it keeps individuals alert and promotes motivation, energy and enthusiasm. Excitement, pleasure or anticipation of a happy event promote arousal and allow us to experience positive stress. Whether you are excited at a happy event or angry following an argument, the body will react in the same way, but it is the individual's reaction that makes it a positive or negative stress reaction.

Our ability to cope with potential challenge or threat will depend on many variable factors including social circumstances, environment and general health. The cause of stress will vary from person to person as it is the individual reaction to threat rather than the threat itself that creates a stress reaction.

A stress reaction is a physical response whereby the body prepares itself to take action. Homeostasis is disrupted as hormones are produced to prepare the body for potential demands.

Negative stress occurs when an individual is faced with a stressor that is unwanted and may cause physical threat creating a dangerous situation that a person would prefer not to cope with.

Short-term stress occurs daily, often as a result of a sudden event such as being asked to speak in front of the class or hearing you have passed your maths test. These everyday events may cause a sudden stress reaction, but the body will quite quickly return to a balanced state and homeostasis will be restored.

Long-term stress occurs when there are one or more stressors that repeatedly present a demand which may exceed a person's capabilities or resources and prevent the return of homeostasis. If this occurs, acute or chronic ill health may follow. People who suffer from stress have a weakened immune system that decreases their resistance to infection and prolongs recovery from illness and trauma.

2 Identifying stressors

Stressors may be defined as stimuli that require a person to make some form of adaptation or adjustment.

Most of our daily life contains stressful events that will cause a physical reaction and the release of hormones to prepare the body for demands and response. Personality, support structures and overall environmental situations will influence the demands made on the individual and determine whether the stressor is seen in a positive or negative manner.

When you reflect on the past 24 hours, are you able to identify 'stressors' that have affected you? Waking up late, spilling a cup of coffee, being on a crowded and noisy bus, these are just a few examples of potential stressors. Stressors are described as being external or internal depending on which environment is creating the stressful stimuli.

External stressors

External stressors relate to the environment around us. Environmental situations, for example a crowded room, constant noise or a very hot or cold classroom, will often cause an element of stress. Social situations also create external stressors, for example if you dislike the company that you are in or you have an argument or disagreement with a family member or work colleague.

The environment around us will have an impact on the stressors and problems that are encountered on a daily basis. External stressors are found in all situations including the following.

Social:

- Overcrowding.
- Antisocial behaviour.
- Conforming to norms and values within society.
- Relationships.

Work:

- Noise and temperature levels.
- Light.
- Restricted movement.
- Low pay.
- Low status.
- Staff shortages.
- Shift work.

- Lack of resources.

- Poor communication channels.

- Work overload.

- Lack of praise.

- Unclear policies or procedures.

- Friction or conflict between staff members.

Home:

- Division of labour.

- Child birth and childcare.

- Domestic labour.

- Lack of recognition for work undertaken.

- Time management.

Internal stressors

Internal stressors are stimuli caused by physiological or psychological stressors from within and may be due to pain or thoughts and feelings. Physiological imbalances in homeostasis will create stress. Pain is a common cause of internal stress. If you suffer from a persistent headache or toothache the stress caused may affect your thoughts and feelings – causing increased anxiety and irritability. In severe illness or trauma, inadequate blood flow to body tissues caused by haemorrhage, burns or dehydration will produce multiple stressors and shock. If shock persists and oxygen levels to organs remain low, cells and organs become damaged and may die.

How you react to a stressor is affected by the situation you are in and your perception of what is happening. If you are in a crowded railway carriage being jostled between fellow passengers you may find crowding a negative stressor, but if you are at a lively party, a crowded room may add to the excitement and you may then perceive crowding as a positive stressor. How people perceive stressors is subjective, as social, environmental, physical and psychological factors must be taken into account for each individual person.

Yerkes-Dodson law

It is difficult to estimate the effects that a stressor will have on daily life as the stress factor may vary depending on the pressures from within ourselves. Stress causes a state of arousal in which the body prepares to meet the challenge of the stressor.

People need stress in the form of arousal in order to perform tasks, but the degree of stress will have an effect on a person's performance. Excessive stress will lead to poor performance and will affect complex tasks to a greater degree than simple ones. If excessive stress continues for a long period, even simple tasks will be affected. The Yerkes-Dodson law (Banyard, 1999) explains that performance will be best when there are moderate levels of arousal and worst when there are very high or very low levels of arousal.

The Yerkes-Dodson law: arousal improves performance up to a point but beyond that point performance will decline

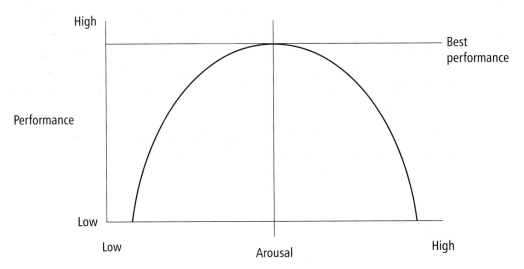

Personal qualities

Personal qualities affect how a person will appraise and respond to stress. If personal qualities include the ability to remain calm and display low levels of anxiety with a high degree of emotional control, stress levels will be low in daily life leading to the possibility of actively seeking activities that have the potential of maximum stress, such as bungee jumping, motor-car racing or mountaineering. If a person finds it difficult to cope with everyday stressors and displays a low degree of emotional control and high anxiety levels, they may respond by seeking minimal stress activities and may be prone to developing phobias or panic attacks.

The different factors involved in determining the effects of a stressor include what a person thinks must be done and what actually can be done in a stressful situation. What can be done will depend on the amount of social support and resources that are believed to be at the person's disposal. If the stressful situation is predictable, a person may have a degree of control and this may relieve some of the stressful qualities of the situation. An ambiguous situation becomes potentially stressful due to loss of control and unpredictability. For example, the unpredictable pressures of finance, planning and keeping the future in-laws content may mar the happy event of a wedding, leading to loss of control and negative stress. If the stressor is one where you are able to cope with the demands made and enjoy the stimulation, the stress is welcome. If you are unable to handle the demands made by the stressor then the stress is unwelcome and detrimental to health.

Occupational stress

The main stressors in life will vary depending on the social environment. As humans, the effect of stressors relates to our instinct for survival. In industrialised countries a major source of stress is work related. Work pressures may include working long hours, meeting deadlines and targets, and having to undertake considerable responsibilities on a daily basis (Spector, 2000). Research (Quine, 1998) shows that healthcare workers appear to be at higher risk of work-related stress than other occupations. Payne and Firth-Cozens (1987) state that this is due to the demands made on healthcare workers who are involved with situations of suffering and death. Further research by Shouksmith and Taylor (1997) states that high stress levels are also due to potential dire consequences if a mistake is made. For healthcare workers occupational stress may be quite considerable.

It is important to be able to recognise the signs and symptoms of stress in order to set about reducing or removing potentially harmful stressors.

3 Signs and symptoms of stress

The signs and symptoms of stress indicate that a person is unable to cope with stressors and that homeostasis is not in balance.

Signs

There are many signs that indicate when a person is suffering from the inability to cope with stress. Signs of stress are visible to the observer. Behavioural and emotional indicators enable you to 'see' that a person is under stress, and these include:

- A low level or lack of concentration.
- Irritability.
- Change in sleep pattern including insomnia.
- Inability to think properly with a tendency for the mind to go blank when trying to recall specific information.
- Shortened attention span.
- Appears disorganised.
- Poor performance in any task undertaken.
- Overindulgence in smoking, alcohol and drugs.
- Daydreaming.
- Accidents at work and home.
- Emotional outbursts.
- Hostile and insulting behaviour.

Symptoms

Symptoms of stress are the physical changes that occur during stressful situations. Although not visible to the observer, the sufferer will complain of various symptoms including:

- Muscle tension and aches.
- Restlessness and the inability to relax.
- Feeling tired and fatigued all of the time.
- Experiencing breathlessness.
- Excessive sweating.
- Clammy hands.

- Dry mouth.

- Feeling of a lump in the throat.

- Nausea.

- Vomiting.

- Diarrhoea.

- Tightness in the chest.

- Frequency of micturition.

- Hot flushes.

- Tooth grinding (bruxism).

- Palpitations.

- Increased pulse rate.

- Raised blood pressure.

- Feeling faint or dizzy.

- Shakiness.

- Feeling bloated or suffering from dyspepsia.

- Nail biting.

Because of the subjective nature of stress it is very difficult to measure exactly how much stress a person is experiencing. The signs and symptoms of stress are caused by physiological responses as the body attempts to maintain home-ostasis.

4 Physiological responses to stress

The body's physical responses to stressors are the same whether the cause is physical (infection, haemorrhage, burns etc.) or psychological (bereavement, emotional, work related etc.). The organ systems involved depend on the nervous and endocrine responses to stress.

Stress and the organ systems involved

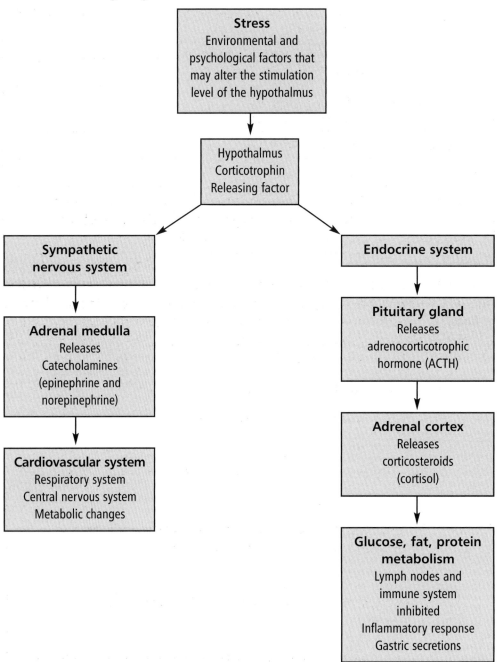

Stress
Environmental and psychological factors that may alter the stimulation level of the hypothalmus

Hypothalmus Corticotrophin Releasing factor

Sympathetic nervous system

Endocrine system

Adrenal medulla
Releases Catecholamines (epinephrine and norepinephrine)

Pituitary gland
Releases adrenocorticotrophic hormone (ACTH)

Cardiovascular system
Respiratory system
Central nervous system
Metabolic changes

Adrenal cortex
Releases corticosteroids (cortisol)

Glucose, fat, protein metabolism
Lymph nodes and immune system inhibited
Inflammatory response
Gastric secretions

In the initial response to stressors the sympathetic branch of the autonomic nervous system and endocrine systems are stimulated to increase the levels of epinephrine (adrenaline) and norepinephrine (noradrenaline) in the bloodstream. The effects of epinephrine and norepinephrine (collectively called the catecholamines) are shown in the table.

Effects of epinephrine and norepinephrine

Organ/system	Effect
Heart	Increased cardiac output
Circulatory system	Dilation of arterioles supplying skeletal muscle, cardiac muscle, liver and adipose tissue
	Constriction of arterioles supplying the gastrointestinal tract, kidney and skin
Respiratory system	Dilation of the bronchus Increased breathing rate
Nervous system	Increased arousal
Eyes	Pupils dilate
Metabolic effects	Glycogen is broken down to form glucose for energy production Release of glucose by the liver to increase blood glucose levels Fat breakdown to release fatty acids for energy production

Catecholamines come into action as the first response to stress, and the endocrine system producing glucocorticoids maintains homeostasis if stress is prolonged. Glucocorticoids take longer to work than the catecholamines but the effect lasts for longer. Glucocorticoid secretion by the adrenal cortex is stimulated by negative feedback.

Glucocorticoid secretion by the adrenal cortex

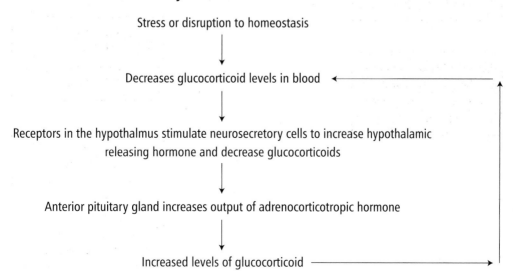

Stress or disruption to homeostasis

Decreases glucocorticoid levels in blood

Receptors in the hypothalmus stimulate neurosecretory cells to increase hypothalamic releasing hormone and decrease glucocorticoids

Anterior pituitary gland increases output of adrenocorticotropic hormone

Increased levels of glucocorticoid

The main actions of the glucocorticoids are shown in the table below.

The main actions of the glucocorticoids

Function	Effect
Carbohydrate metabolism	Inhibits glucose intake in tissues except for the brain and heart. This increases blood glucose levels
	Stimulates glucose production from stored glycogen, proteins and fat
	Enhances the effect of catecholamines
Protein metabolism	Breaks down protein molecules
	Depresses protein synthesis
	Increases production of urea
Immune system	Decreases the mass of lymphatic tissue
	Decreases the number of circulating lymphocytes and other white blood cells
Inflammatory response	Reduces inflammation
Other functions	Promotes gastric secretions – the cause of peptic ulcers
	Increases urinary output
	May enhance learning

The effects continue with raised stress levels and may cause damage to the heart and cardiovascular system if epinephrine and cortisol levels remain high. If the immune system is suppressed for a prolonged period of time the body will become increasingly susceptible to disease and illness (McEwen, 1998).

Following illness or trauma, the physiological response to stressors is controlled by negative and positive feedback systems. In severe cases of trauma the disruption to homeostasis will affect all organs of the body. If the cardiovascular system fails to deliver adequate oxygen and nutrients to the organs and cells, shock will occur. The severity of shock will vary depending on the cause. Symptoms of shock include:

- A systolic blood pressure of below 90 mm Hg.

- Rapid, weak pulse and rapid heart rate – caused by the involvement of the sympathetic nervous system and increased levels of epinephrine.

- Cold, clammy, pale skin – vasoconstriction of blood vessels to peripheral organs. Sweating increased due to sympathetic nervous system involvement.

- Reduced urine output – increased levels of aldosterone and antidiuretic hormone.

- Nausea and vomiting – vasoconstriction of vessels supplying the digestive system.

- Confusion and/or reduced level of consciousness – reduced oxygen supply to the brain.

If the state of shock occurs, medical intervention will be required to assist in reversing the effects of positive feedback and to restore homeostasis.

5 Models of stress

There are different ways of studying stressors and coping mechanisms. The following are the three main categories used to approach the study of stress. Stress as a stimulus:

- Stress is viewed as an independent variable.

- The stress is caused by an event or circumstance and the stressors are described in terms of threats or pressures from the environment.

Stress as a response:

- Stress is viewed as a dependent variable.

- Stressors cause a physiological or psychological reaction in response to a potential threat.

Stress as an intervening variable:

- Stress is viewed as the result of the imbalance caused by stress and the individual's ability to cope.

- The demands made by results of a stressor will depend on perceived or actual resources available to cope with the demand. The resources include biological, psychological and social factors.

Models of stress are the different approaches to the study of stress.

The stimulus-based model

This model is based on stressors as external or environmental factors that provoke a response or a series of responses. These responses are known as strains.

External stressor	The individual
Stress	Strain
Cause	*Effect*
Noise	Muscle tension
Poor lighting	Headache
Conflict	Depression
Physical illness	Anxiety/fatigue

The effects of stress may create a variety of strains. Loud noise may produce the strain of irritation that in turn may result in a raised pulse rate and blood pressure. Holmes and Rahe's social readjustment rating scale (see topic 6) is an example of viewing stress by way of a stimulus-based model. Although this model examines stress as an external factor that impinges on an individual, it does not make allowances for individual responses.

The response-based model

In this model, stress is described as the changes that take place within an individual as a response to potentially damaging or damaging external or internal stressors that create demands on the body. In this model any stimulus that produces a 'stress response' must be a stressor. When faced with stress the body will undergo a range of physiological, thought and behavioural changes.

In 1932 Walter Cannon described the physiological reaction to threat as the 'fight or flight' response. This response is the immediate action taken when a threat is present, allowing a person to fight the threat or escape from it. The threat may come from a variety of emotions or physical activities called the 'E' situations – exercise, emergency, excitement or embarrassment.

When the fight or flight response is triggered increased levels of epinephrine and norepinephrine are released into the bloodstream preparing the body to make the appropriate physical response. If you are involved in a very stressful situation, such as an accident or a confrontation, there will be an immediate physiological response; muscles will tense, colour drains from the face, breathing becomes faster and a knotting sensation develops in the stomach, which indicates that your body is preparing to defend itself by fighting or running away. The response to such an event happens very quickly, but even if the situation resolves the response may take a long time to subside. The initial recovery response may include shaking, crying and weakness. Recovery may be prolonged if anxiety or a perceived threat of associated situations remains and this may have long-term consequences on health.

Hans Selye (1956) used Cannon's work to produce a model of stress that looked at the explanation for stress-related illness. Selye experimented with laboratory rats to show that regardless of the type of stressor used, the rats all developed similar physiological reactions. The laboratory observations led Selye to develop the General Adaptation Syndrome that demonstrated how stress might lead to poor health.

The General Adaptation Syndrome suggests that there are three stages in the response to stressful situations:

1. Alarm reaction: this mobilises the body's resources but it cannot be sustained for long periods.

2. Stage of resistance: the body adapts to the stressor. Arousal levels decline but remain raised above homeostatic levels. There are few 'signs' of stress, but the ability to resist new stressors is impaired. The individual becomes vulnerable to raised blood pressure etc.

3. Exhaustion: The body is depleted of energy reserves. If stress continues, disease, damage or death may occur as adaptation is no longer possible.

In this model of stress the response of the body is to restore homeostasis as quickly as possible.

The main weakness of this theory is that it looks at the biological response but does not take into account any psychological or behavioural variables.

The transactional model

Lazarus and Folkman (1984) identified the experience of stress as a series of events in which each stressor is appraised. The first reaction to a stressor is the primary appraisal to allow the person to judge if the stressor is positive (good), neutral (causing little effect) or negative (harmful). If the primary appraisal judges the stressor to be harmful, a second appraisal is made to determine if coping abilities and support/resources are sufficient to overcome the potential harm. If the stressor is sufficient to cause harm then stress will be evident as physiological, emotional and behavioural changes occur.

In this model the individual plays an important part in moderating the stress response by taking into account memories of relevant previous events. This is called cognitive appraisal. It allows a person to evaluate the degree of threat or harm that is occurring or is likely to occur. In the first instance the person must evaluate how much harm has occurred, what further harm may occur and the degree of challenge the stressor demands. Then judgement must be made on how the person believes they can cope – this will depend on their health and state of mind. The physiological changes that occur during stress may be modified by the person's perceptions of circumstances.

The transactional model makes the point that what is threatening and stressful to one person may not be so for everyone because personal characteristics and experiences are taken into account. Personal qualities and the feeling and thought of control or predictability as well as the relationship with the environment may moderate the stress response.

This model includes the physiological and psychological homeostasis and accounts for individual response to similar stressors. The transactional model can be applied to major physical, environmental or psychological trauma and is often used in healthcare settings. By understanding the effects of stressors on an individual basis, healthcare workers are able to respond to clients' fears and anxieties with a higher degree of empathy.

The theories and models of stress may be used as a tool when measuring stress response.

6 Measuring stress

Because of the subjective nature of stress it is very difficult to measure exactly how much stress a person is experiencing. Psychologists have devised different scales in an attempt to measure stress levels.

Holmes and Rahe (1967) developed the Social Readjustment Rating Scale following data collected from over 5000 patients. The ratings on the scale relate to the increased problems with ill health or accidents following social readjustment after a major life event.

Social Readjustment Rating Scale

Life event	Mean value
1. Death of a spouse	100
2. Divorce	73
3. Marital separation	65
4. Jail term	63
5. Death of a close member of the family	63
6. Personal injury or illness	53
7. Marriage	50
8. Loss of job	47
9. Marital reconciliation	45
10. Retirement	45
11. Major health changes of family member	44
12. Pregnancy	40
13. Sex difficulties	39
14. Gaining a new family member	39
15. Business readjustment	39
16. Change in financial state	38
17. Death of a close friend	37
18. Changing jobs	36
19. Change in the number of arguments with spouse	35
20. Mortgage over $10,000 (today's value $100,000 (approx. £57,500))	31
21. Foreclosure on a mortgage or a loan	29
22. Change in responsibilities at work	29
23. Son or daughter leaving home	29
24. Trouble with the in-laws	28
25. Outstanding personal achievement	26
26. Spouse beginning or stopping work	26
27. Begin or end school	26
28. Change in living conditions	25

Life event	Mean value
29. Revision of personal habits	24
30. Trouble with employer	23
31. Change in work hours or commitments	20
32. Change in residence	20
33. Change in schools	20
34. Change in recreation	19
35. Change in church activities	19
36. Change in social activities	18
37. Mortgage or loan less than $10,000 (today's value $100,000 (approx. £57,500))	17
38. Change in sleeping patterns	16
39. Change in number of family social events	15
40. Change in eating habits	15
41. Vacation	13
42. Christmas	12
43. Minor violation of the law	11

Source: Holmes and Rahe (1967)

Point value is given to express the severity of an event that has occurred during the previous months. If a person's score is above 200 they are at risk of developing a stress-related illness and urgent measures should be undertaken to reduce stress. People who experience life events with a high mean value tend to have poorer health.

This rating scale is rather out of date as it does not take into account social change that has occurred in recent years, in particular the changing roles of women. It views all events as stressful, but does not acknowledge positive stress. The scale has been criticised as it does not include factors of poverty or racism that may affect low social economic or minority groups. However, the Social Readjustment Rating Scale is still used as an approach to measuring stress as it does give an indication of the types of stressors a person has experienced.

Many people suffer from stress without experiencing major life events. The degree of stress suffered by a person will therefore also depend on stressors encountered on a day-to-day basis. Lazarus, Kanner and Folkman (1980) researched daily 'hassles' and the effect they have on stress levels.

Daily hassles will cause physiological and physical symptoms of stress to occur. The effects that daily hassles have on stress levels will vary depending on the social support available. Kanner *et al.* noted that if people were to experience uplifts (i.e. positive events) they would suffer less from the effects of daily hassles.

The hassles scale

This scale shows hassles that are commonly experienced by college students.

The hassles may occur several times within a month. The hassles are circled and rated as to the severity of stress caused. 1 = somewhat severe, 2 = moderately severe, 3 = extremely severe. Students who experience a high number of daily hassles during a one-month period tend to indicate poorer health

1. Conflicts with partner/spouse
2. Being let down or disappointed by friends
3. Too many things to do at once
4. Getting lower grades than you hoped for
5. Separation from people you care about
6. Inadequate leisure time
7. Loneliness
8. Dissatisfaction with your athletic skills
9. Not enough time for sleep
10. Disliking your studies

Source: Kanner et al.(1981)

Uplifts scale

This scale shows events that are positive and make a person feel good. The rating is the same as the hassles list and is measured over a one-month period. A high frequency of uplifting experiences during a one-month period tends to indicate better psychological and physical health.

1. Saving money
2. Relating well with partner/spouse
3. Socialising
4. Reading
5. Shopping
6. Spending time with family
7. Sex
8. Growing confidence
9. Doing volunteer work
10. Being a good listener

Source: Kanner et al. (1981)

Perceived stress

People have the ability to evaluate experiences of stress in different ways and this makes it difficult to judge if a stressor will cause harm. Often a person's perception of a stressor will affect the physical response to stress.

The attitudes, needs, past experiences, personality traits, age, gender and education of an individual will influence their actual ability to cope. If they have an apparent ability to cope with the perceived demand, the response may be the strain of coping or not coping. If they are able to cope then the actual demand made by the stressor will be met. If they are unable to cope, symptoms of stress will develop. The person will then need to explore the situation to re-evaluate the apparent ability to cope with perceived demand, taking into account environmental and social factors. If a person believes that they have support from outside agencies, including family and friends, the success of perceived ability to cope is increased.

The following is a mother's account of children's swimming lessons:

> The first session of swimming lessons took place after school. A frantic dash from school to the leisure centre left only minutes to spare. The changing room was overcrowded, noisy and hot with small single cubicles in a unisex area. The layout of the changing rooms allowed children to run and hide around the cubicle blocks with their heads narrowly missing the open metal locker doors. The swimming instructor was less than complimentary about the children's swimming abilities. The shower facilities were designed so that to extract the child from the shower the parent had no alternative but to get wet. Only one child could be helped at one time due to the size of the changing cubicles, leaving the other to drop dry clothes onto the wet floor or disappear into another unknown cubicle.

Control was lost, stress levels rose, and signs and symptoms of stress were present.

At the next lesson signs and symptoms of stress became apparent on entering the leisure complex. This exaggerated the stressors of heat, noise and overcrowding. Soon the mere thought of swimming lessons produced palpitations, muscle tension and increased respiratory rate.

Swimming lessons became the main stressor of the week. Action was taken to reduce the effects: sleeveless tops to combat the heat, and strict rules of conduct were issued to the children. Then friendships were established with other parents who also battled through the stressful event of swimming lessons. Humour of the situation was seen. Although swimming lessons remained a potential stressor, the physiological and psychological effects were greatly reduced as perceived stress was reduced.

Physiological measures of stress

Physiological measures of stress are used to measure heart rate, blood pressure, respiratory rate and skin conductance (a measure of sweating). Biological measures of hormones in the blood or urine are also used to indicate stress levels.

Experiments to quantify stress using physiological measures have limitations as the environment and equipment needed to record the body's functions may in themselves cause stress. White-coat hypertension may occur when a person becomes stressed when they have their blood pressure recorded in a clinical setting. Age, gender, weight, physical fitness and general health must also be taken into account.

Biological measures are more reliable as raised levels of corticosteroids and catecholamines are found in individuals who have experienced stressful situations or are suffering from long-term stress. However, blood tests may increase stress levels and they are expensive to carry out.

Therefore, individual reactions are a variable factor in measuring stress and this must be taken into account when interpreting the results.

7 How stress affects health

In modern-day society, with its rapid pace of life, people are confronted with long periods of stress resulting in an increase of stress-related illness.

Stress causes illness in the following ways:

- Directly by reducing the body's ability to fight illness by creating an imbalance in homeostasis.

- Indirectly by leading the person to adopt an unhealthy lifestyle.

The response to stress is controlled mainly by the hypothalamus. The hypothalmic-releasing hormones stimulate the anterior pituitary gland to secrete ACTH, human growth hormone and thyroid-stimulating hormone. The hormones help to break down glycogen to glucose to supply additional adenosine triphosphate (ATP), the energy-carrying molecule. If exposure to stress is prolonged, the high levels of cortisol and hormones will affect the body by causing wasting of muscles, suppression of the immune system, ulceration of the gastrointestinal tract and failure of pancreatic beta cells. People who suffer from prolonged effects of stress have a greater risk of developing chronic disease or may die prematurely.

Glaser and Kiecolt-Glaser (1994) state that people who suffer from long-term stress have an increased incidence of experiencing associated illness and disease.

Stress-induced illness is a controversial subject and only with the knowledge of causal pathways have some disorders been accepted as having stress as an underlying cause. Illnesses that have been generally accepted to be stress related are:

- Gastrointestinal disorders – duodenal and stomach ulcers.

- Rheumatoid disease – immune response.

- Asthma, hay fever – abnormal immune response.

- Eclampsia and renal disease – secondary to hypertension.

- Eczema and other atopic skin diseases – immune response.

- Cancer.

- Diabetes mellitus.

- Multiple sclerosis, rheumatoid arthritis – autoimmune disorder.

- Cardiovascular disease – angina, myocardial infarct – precipitated by hypertension and high cholesterol levels.

- Myalgic encephalomyelitis (ME) – immune response.

- Mental illness – from signs of anxiety to severe mental illness.

Other possible illnesses that may be stress related are:

- Shingles – immune response.

- Irritable bowel syndrome.

- Urinary incontinence.

- Migraine.

- Chronic headache.

- Bronchial asthma.

- Cancer of the uterus (post menopause).

There are many indirect effects of stress on health caused by changes in behaviour.

Changes in behaviour caused by stress

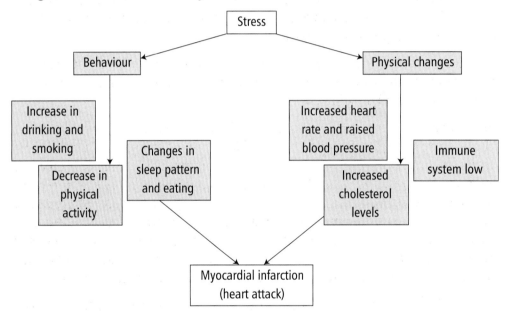

An increased risk of a myocardial infarction, particularly in people over the age of 40 years, is thought to be due to:

- Stress – physical reaction or response to stressful event/s.

- Fat being released into the bloodstream as the body responds to stress. This is caused by increased flow of epinephrine. The fat cells (particularly around the stomach area) will respond to increases in epinephrine by releasing fatty acids into the bloodstream.

- The liver converting the fatty acid into triglycerides and then into low-density lipoprotein.

- High levels of lipoproteins, associated with the formation of atherosclerotic plaques in the coronary arteries. The plaques are lesions that form on the endothelial lining of the artery due to various causes including: high levels of lipoproteins, prolonged high blood pressure, cytomegalovirus (herpes virus), high carbon monoxide levels (cigarette smoking) and diabetes mellitus.

- An increase in triglycerides, which may disrupt the blood sugar levels and cause a rise in insulin. Raised insulin levels stimulate the sympathetic nervous system and blood pressure is increased.

- High blood pressure, which may cause an unstable atherosclerotic plaque to rupture. The body will stimulate the clotting process to repair the damaged artery, but during this process the diameter of the artery will be reduced, blood flow will be impeded and obstruction of blood flow will lead to depletion of oxygen supplies to the cardiac muscle. The muscle area supplied with blood from the obstructed artery will die – a myocardial infarct – if blood flow is not restored immediately.

How a person manages their own stress appears to have a direct link with general well-being. It is the interaction between stress and the individual that will determine how a potential stressor is interpreted.

For example, as a student you may find the process of sitting exams or making presentations stressful; emotions such as anxiety and fear have a negative effect and may lead to behavioural changes.

During exam time it is probable that your blood pressure will become slightly raised as levels of epinephrine and cortisol increase. Suppression of the immune system will decrease your white cell count. The risk of infections are increased. Wounds will take longer to heal and you may take longer to recover from a common cold. In addition to this your lifestyle may change to make time for studies. Lack of physical exercise and staying up late to revise will disrupt your sleep pattern and you may turn to an unhealthy diet to keep you going! Excessive cups of tea or coffee, high-sugar snacks, convenience foods, smoking and alcohol will have a direct negative impact on your health thus increasing the stress levels.

The associated physiological processes that make stress a risk to homeostasis may be a direct response or an indirect response because of changes in behaviour patterns linked to coping with stress. During revision time you may find that suddenly small matters become much more stressful than usual. The television blaring, the children wanting constant attention, a partner asking when dinner will be ready – any of these may suddenly become a huge issue. Arguments may follow, causing even higher levels of stress.

Burnout

Routine stresses caused by constant pressure at home or in the workplace may lead to feelings of frustration, tiredness and apathy.

If stress continues then emotional exhaustion occurs and the person will suffer 'burnout'. Cognitive skills will be affected and they will no longer be able to cope with the demands being made and their work will suffer. Difficulty in concentrating on tasks, and poor memory and attention are signs of burnout.

Burnout is common amongst health professionals and other caring or helping professions such as police officers, fire fighters and social workers. According to Quine (1998) the most stressful demands made on employees within the National Health Service were role overload, responsibility for others, demands made by management (organisational demands), uncertainty of role and problems in the work environment. A report by Allen (2001) shows that the main reasons that nurses gave for stress were:

- Staffing of busy wards.

- Worries about the competency levels of staff.

- Long hours.

- Recruitment and retention of staff.

- Cleanliness of wards.

- Stress from other healthcare professionals.

- Not feeling valued by the organisation.

- Communication.

Stress is the most common reason for sick leave within the National Health Service (HSE, 2001).

Behaviour patterns

Although stress is hard to define and stressors are varied, the reaction to stress may be linked to individual personality types.

In 1959 Freidman and Roseman completed a 12-year longitudinal study investigating behaviour patterns relating to the psychological influences of stress. They established that there were two distinct behaviour patterns, pattern A and pattern B.

Pattern A behaviour was described as:

- Intense sustained drive to achieve personal goals.

- Eagerness and tendency to compete in all situations.

- A persistent desire for recognition and advancement.

- Continuous involvement in several activities at once, that are subject to deadlines.

- Habitual tendencies to rush to finish activities.

- Extraordinary mental and physical alertness.

Pattern B behaviour was described as:

- The opposite of pattern A, with a relative absence of drive, ambition, urgency, desire to complete, or involvement with deadlines.

Pattern A behaviour personalities are more likely to suffer from symptoms of stress including headaches, muscle tension and illness. There may also be potential problems with interpersonal relationships and a feeling of discontentment with life.

Pattern B behaviour personalities tend to enjoy better health and feelings of satisfaction with life.

When related to coronary heart disease, Ragland and Brand (1988) discovered a difference in survival rate following myocardial infarction (MI) of pattern A and B behaviour personalities. Twenty-four hours following an MI, pattern A had a greater survival rate than pattern B. This is possibly due to the fact that pattern A was able to significantly modify their behaviour and in doing so greatly reduced their stress levels.

Post traumatic stress disorder

High-stress, dramatic events may have long-term effects on health. Post traumatic stress disorder (PTSD) was first recognised as a real and serious condition in 1980 following an article in the 3rd edition of the *Diagnostic and Statistical Manual of Mental Disorders* of the American Psychiatric Association.

The symptoms of PTSD include:

- Recurrent flashbacks.

- Active avoidance of thoughts, feelings or similar situations associated with the dramatic event.

- Increased arousal leading to signs of stress.

PTSD may be experienced immediately after the event or in some cases months or years later.

8 Coping mechanisms, responses and strategies

'Adaptation' is the term used when physiological responses are used to control homeostasis during illness or trauma. The psychological or behavioural responses are known as coping mechanisms. In many illnesses or during trauma, both adaptation and coping responses are required to restore homeostasis.

To help cope with anxiety and other stress-related emotions, unconscious defence mechanisms will be employed to act as protection against the pain of life experiences. Common forms of defence mechanism are:

- Identification – a person will unconsciously copy the behaviour or mannerisms of a person they admire or envy. This may occur when a newly qualified nurse is placed in charge of a ward for the first time.

- Repression – an unconscious refusal to come to terms with change or problems, keeping thoughts that might provoke anxiety out of the conscious mind. This may lead to a 'forgotten' doctors' appointment as the thought of a potentially stressful situation is repressed from conscious thought.

- Denial – denying any changes have occurred and behaving accordingly to escape from stress. If a client is told they have a terminal illness they may then proceed to act as if nothing is seriously wrong.

- Regression – returning to previous behaviour, in extreme cases regression to childhood behaviour.

- Introjection – if a threat is made the individual may internalise the attitudes of those making the threats. Children often do this by pretending to be the person who threatens them in order to cope with their fear.

- Projection – attributing our own unacceptable behaviours, thoughts and feelings to another person. Blaming someone else for an incident; in the workplace this is quite common.

- Reaction formation – turning feelings (love) into the reverse (hate).

- Displacement – this involves redirecting negative feelings and actions away from the source to a safer target. (If your boss shouts at you, instead of shouting back you go home and shout at the children.)

- Sublimation – to keep thoughts away the individual becomes obsessed with work or takes up a new hobby or sport.

- Rationalisation – this involves making excuses or justifying a situation in order to limit feelings, responsibility or disappointment. (For example, 'I have been too busy to study so I know that I am going to fail this assignment'.)

Problem and emotion-focused strategies

Accepting that stress is an essential element of life is the first step in coping with it. There are as many ways of coping with stress as there are ways of experiencing stress. The strategies used to deal with stress are often divided into two groups, as shown in the figure.

Strategies used to deal with stress

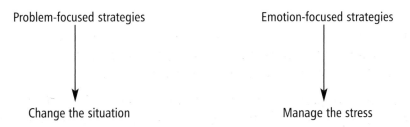

Problem-focused strategies   Emotion-focused strategies

Change the situation   Manage the stress

Source: Lazarus and Folkman, 1980

Problem-focused strategies

In problem-focused strategies stress is managed by trying to confront and change the stressor. It is an effective coping mechanism as it involves constructive ways of solving problems. The problems may be solved in a number of ways.

Active coping:

- Concentrating efforts on problem.

- Making a plan of action.

- Taking direct action.

- Seeking information and advice.

- Seeking support and guidance for emotional support.

- Learning from the experience.

Emotion-focused strategies

Emotion-focused strategies cope with stress by managing the emotional effects of stress.

Distancing:

- Refusing to look at the problem seriously.

- Pretending there is no problem.

- Trying to forget the problem.

Self-controlling:

- Keeping feelings to oneself.

- Keeping feelings from others.

Escape, avoidance:

- Wishing the problem would go away.

- Hoping a miracle will happen.

- Trying to improve feelings by eating, drinking etc.

Emotion-focused strategies are associated with negative adjustment to prevent a person from understanding and coming to terms with problems. The use of denial may have a serious impact on health if a person delays seeking medical care for potentially life-threatening conditions.

In both strategies the resources and social support available will affect the outcome and effectiveness of coping mechanisms.

Resources for coping

Resources for coping may be physical, psychological or materialistic. There are many areas from which to obtain resources, including the following.

Material resources – wealth to buy goods, including:

- Healthcare.

- Safe environment.

- Warm and relaxing environment.

- Food.

- Medicines.

Physical resources:

- Strength or hardiness.

- Attractiveness.

- Health.

Intra-personal:

- Inner strength.

- Personality.

Educational:

- Knowledge – to moderate behaviour and reduce the risks.

Cultural:

- Social setting.
- Religion.

Social support

Perhaps the most important resource in coping mechanisms is the amount of social support an individual believes they have. Social support may be given by family, friends, fellow workers, religious or social groups. The knowledge that support and help is available if required will be a useful tool in emotion- and problem-focused strategies.

Cohen and Wills (1985) identified social support as follows.

Esteem support:

- The support that allows an individual to feel valued and respected by others. This raises self esteem.

Informational support:

- Useful information may be gained from social contacts.
- Professional advice.

Instrumental support:

- Financial support.
- Material resources.
- Appropriate tangible support.

Social companionship:

- Spending time and being able to talk to others.
- The sense of belonging.

Social support may be actual support or perceived support. If an individual perceives that support will be given if needed, they will be able to predict an outcome. This may help in determining what coping strategies to use. Some research shows that perceived support is a stronger predictor of well-being than received support (Cohen and Wills, 1985).

The value of social support has been identified as a factor in survival and recovery rates following illness or trauma. Kulik and Mahler (1989) carried out a study to examine the link between speed of recovery of male clients following coronary bypass surgery and the social support received from their partners. They concluded that receiving a high level of support was beneficial, and clients with support requested less pain-relief medication and recovery times were reduced. Clients who had an unsupportive partner had a slower recovery rate with their hospital stay being extended for an average of 1.26 days. Schwarzer and Leppin (1992) support this hypothesis in their study which showed that twice as many single people die from coronary heart disease as married people. Williams *et al.* (1992) provide statistics to indicate that clients with heart disease have a lower mortality rate if they are married or have a partner.

Social support is difficult to define as there are many variables that must be considered in each individual situation. Positive social relationships may enhance health and well-being by encouraging and promoting healthy behaviour. Social support may also provide a buffer from everyday stress providing a reserve and resource that blunts the effects of stress. Buffering helps to protect individuals from the negative effects of high stress and therefore has a positive effect on health (Wills, 1984).

Social support may influence the appraisal of stressors and the coping strategies to be employed. Social support will also have an effect on physiological reactions to stress. Research has shown that people who have a large social network are less susceptible to the common cold (Cohen *et al.*, 1997). Individuals who have effective social support demonstrate the following physiological signs and symptoms during periods of high stress:

- Lower pulse and blood pressure.
- Increased white cell count.
- Greater natural killer-cell activity.
- Lower levels of epinephrine, norepinephrine and cortisol.

There is occasionally a negative aspect of social support. For example, if a child has asthma the family may respond by overprotective behaviour, which may lead to the child becoming stressed due to over-concern and this manifests itself in an increase in asthmatic symptoms. The social support may also reinforce behaviour associated with illness leading to a prolonged period of ill health.

Problem and emotion-focused strategies may be used for different situations and a combination of the strategies, resources and social support help to form an effective coping mechanism. The outcome of coping strategies will lead to the individual being able to cope and carry on with life, or leave them with feelings of distress and possible long-term illness.

Psychotherapeutic drugs

Drug therapy is available to reduce the physiological effects of severe or chronic stress. The drugs affect the autonomic nervous system and have central-muscle relaxant properties. Side effects of the drugs may include drowsiness, sedation and unsteadiness, with occasional adverse reactions including hypotension, gastrointestinal upsets, visual disturbances and changes in libido. In some cases abnormal psychological reactions of aggressive outbursts, confusion, excitement, and depression with suicidal tendencies have been reported. Drug therapy should only be given as a short-term measure as clients may become dependent on the medication. Withdrawal from the drugs may cause symptoms such as depression, irritability, nervousness, diarrhoea, insomnia and sweating. Drug therapy reduces the signs and symptoms of stress but does not help to identify the stressors or improve long-term coping abilities.

9 Techniques to improve coping strategies

There are several therapies that may be used to help individuals improve coping abilities and reduce stress.

Biofeedback

Biofeedback is a relaxation technique that aims to give a person feedback on how psychological states may influence their physiological responses. Clients are attached to a monitor that displays pulse rate, blood pressure and muscle tension and they are able to learn how to use emotions and feelings to control physiological reactions that are not under conscious control. During times of stress the clients are encouraged to use visual or auditory cues to help take control of body responses and to reduce stress.

Used with deep relaxation techniques, biofeedback has been found to reduce symptoms associated with chronic headaches (Budzynski *et al.*, 1970) and irritable bowel syndrome (Kiecolt-Glaser *et al.*, 1986).

Imagery

Tension-reducing imagery practice (TRIP) technique involves educating an individual to use mental imagery to relieve stress or control pain. The individual must use breathing exercises to control respiratory rates and then imagine a scene that is unconnected to or incompatible with the pain or stress, for example standing on a beach and imagining all of the associated sights, sounds and tastes. This strategy appears to be effective, but the reasons why or how imagery works are still not clear. Imagery is often combined with relaxation techniques to promote deep muscle relaxation.

Relaxation techniques

Relaxation techniques aim to develop strategies to lower a person's state of arousal. This technique includes controlling breathing rate and depth to reduce arousal levels and promote relaxation. This technique may be useful to control high levels of anxiety or low-level pain. Relaxation will decrease the muscle tension associated with pain, reduce blood pressure and lower the heart rate.

Meditation

Meditation is a technique where a person assumes a comfortable position to relax their body, eyes closed in an attempt to focus on a single thought. A single-syllable word or mantra may be verbalised or silently repeated. Wallace and

Fisher (1987) found that meditation reduces oxygen consumption and induces electrical activity in the brain indicative of a calm mental state.

Cognitive-behavioural therapies

All therapies that focus on challenging individuals' beliefs on how they perceive stressors and developing coping skills are termed cognitive-behavioural therapies. The aim is to reduce the negative emotions associated with stressors and implement a specific plan to cope with stressful situations. The therapies are useful in many chronic illnesses to reduce the symptoms of anxiety, pain, raised blood pressure and depression. Therapies are also used for intervention, to assist in lowering stress and anxiety in clients with cancer, asthma and epilepsy.

Stress inoculation

Stress inoculation is a technique used to prepare a person for stressful events by:

- Conceptualisation – thinking about the stressor. This is learning to identify and express fears and feelings about individual stressors. The person is educated about stress and stressors.

- Skill acquisition and rehearsal – how to act when the stressor occurs. Instruction is given on behavioural skills and relaxation techniques to be used when faced with stressors.

- Application and follow through – practice in how to act when a stressor occurs. The person is subjected to stressors in order to prepare them for real-life situations.

Humour

Humour has been shown to improve functions of the immune system, producing increased numbers of natural killer cells and lower levels of cortisol (Lefcourt *et al.*, 1990). Humour allows a person to cope with stressors by distracting them from the stressor and allowing them personal control over the situation.

Alternative therapies

There are a vast array of alternative therapies such as acupuncture, aromatherapy and homeopathy that are used as coping strategies for stress. Although not scientifically based, alternative therapies may be useful in helping individuals to improve their coping abilities.

10 Controlling physiological effects of stress

Stress management techniques are used in an attempt to reduce or prevent stressors that have harmful effects on the body, causing an imbalance in home-ostasis. To effectively relieve or control stress that causes harmful physiological reactions, the biopsychosocial responses should be taken into account.

Biological responses

Controlling biological responses requires a person to become aware of their body: enhanced body awareness. It requires a person to be in harmony with their body and conscious of changes in muscle tension and breathing rhythms and have the ability to restore homeostasis by:

- Relaxation and meditation.
- Breathing exercises.
- Biofeedback.

Psychological factors

To assist a person in recognising what they perceive as a stressor and/or help to modify type A behaviour, the following techniques may be useful in reducing stress levels:

- Stress inoculation.
- Assertiveness training.
- Cognitive behaviour therapy.

Sociological factors

To assist in coping with stress the following sociological factors must be taken into account:

- Healthy diet – a nutritional and well-balanced diet.
- Physical exercise – sustained exercise can reduce depression and boost feelings of self-esteem through the release of ß-endorphins, natural opiates that can trigger the same feeling of euphoria as drugs such as opium.
- Finding alternatives to harmful coping behaviours such as smoking, drinking alcohol, excessive amounts of caffeine, drug and solvent abuse.
- Time management strategies – setting realistic goals.
- Social support – emotional, financial and advice. The quality of social support will vary depending on culture and gender.

Stress and well-being

In all aspects of healthcare, direct and indirect stressors are shown to cause a disturbed homeostasis that is identified via imbalances in psychophysical body responses. The effects of stress occur when the stress threshold is superseded.

The integration of sociology, psychology and physiology help healthcare workers investigate stress to gain an understanding of the effects of multiple cumulative stressors and stress-related conditions. Individual care and a holistic approach to treatment is required when planning a multi-dimensional approach to stress management.

Lifestyles and behaviours such as eating, drinking, smoking and exercise have a major impact on the average person's health. Lifestyle choices, stress management and general outlook on life are under our control. People who have an optimistic outlook on life, who believe they have control within their lives and who expect to be healthy will generally remain healthy even if subjected to intense stress. People who have a pessimistic outlook and expect to become ill generally experience more illness after only moderate stress. This is called the self-fulfilling prophecy – what we expect to happen tends to happen.

Health promotion for healthcare workers and clients is a growing area of healthcare work. Many organisations, including the National Health Service, provide in-service training on stress management to employees. Stress management aims to inform people of strategies for relaxation and techniques that will prevent high stress levels from occurring. However, this is a difficult task if conditions of employment include low pay, low status, shift work, staff shortages and lack of resources.

It must be remembered that stress is needed to help us survive. We would be a very apathetic and dull society if we lived in a 'stress free' environment. However, an awareness of well-being and promotion of healthy lifestyles will allow us to improve coping strategies and hopefully reduce the number of stress-related illnesses and associated diseases that are becoming an increasing health problem in industrialised nations.

Further reading

Bahrke, M. W. and Morgan, W. P. (1978) Anxiety reduction following exercise and meditation. *Cognitive therapy and research*, **2**, 627–635.

Fontana, D. (1989) *Managing Stress: The British Psychological Society*. Routledge, London.

Freidman, M. and Roseman, R. H. (1985) *Type A Behaviour and Your Heart*. Knopf, New York.

Gross, R., McLiveen, R. and Coolican, H. (2000) *Psychology: A New Introduction for AS Level*. Hodder and Stoughton, Wiltshire.

Hodgkinson, P. E. and Stewart, M. (1991) *Coping with a Catastophe*. Routledge, London.

Johnston, M., Wright, S. and Weinman, J. (1995) *Measures in Health Psychology*. NFER-Nelson, Windsor.

Manuch, S. B., Kaplan, J. R. Adams, M. R. and Clarkson, T. B. (1989) Behaviourally elicited heart rate re-activity and atherosclerosis in female cynomologus monkeys (macaca fascicularis). *Journal of Psychosomatic Medicine*, **51**, 306–318.

Pitts, M. and Phillips, K. (eds) (1991) *The Psychology of Health*. Routledge, London.

Sanderson, C. A. (2004) *Health Psychology*. John Wiley & Sons, Crawfordsville.

Skinner, B. F. (1995) *Percieved Control, Motivation and Coping*. Sage, London.

Wycherley, R. (1991) *Living Skills Handbook*. Outset Publishing, London.

References

Allen, I. (2001) *Stress among ward sisters and staff nurses*. NHS Executive Report.

American Psychiatric Association (1980) *Diagnostic and Statistical Manual of Mental Disorders*, 3rd edn. Washington DC.

Banyard, P. (1999) *Applying Psychology to Health*. Hodder & Stoughton, Wiltshire.

Budzynski, T. H., Stoyva, J. and Adler, C. S. (1970) Feedback-induced muscle relaxation: Application to tension headache. *Journal of Behaviour Therapy and Experimental Psychiatry*, **1**, 205–211.

Cannon, W. B. (1932) *The Wisdom of the Body*. Norton, New York.

Cohen, S. (1988) Psychosocial models of the role of social support in the etiology of physical disease. *Health Psychology*, **7**, 269–297.

Cohen, S., Doyle, W. J. Skoner, D. P., Rabin B. S. and Gwaltney, J. M. (1997) Social ties and susceptibility to the common cold. *Journal of the American Medical Association*, **277**, 1940–1944.

Cohen, S. and Wills, T. A. (1985) 'Stress, social support, and the buffering hypothesis. *Psychology Bulletin*, **98**, 310–357.

Engel, G. L. (1980) ;The clinical application of the biopsychosocial model. *American Journal of Psychiatry*, **137**, 535–544.

Friedman, M. and Roseman, R. H. (1959) Association of specific overt pattern with blood and cardiovascular findings. *Journal of the American Medical Association*, **169**, 1286–1296.

Glaser, R. and Kiecolt-Glaser, J. K. (1994) *Handbook of Stress and Immunity*. Academic Press, San Diego, CA.

Health and Safety Executive (2001) *Work Related Stress Factors. The Whitehall Study CRR 266/2000*. HSE Books, London.

Holmes, T. H. and Rahe, R. H. (1967) The social readjustment rating scale. *Journal of Psychosomatic Research*, **11**, 213–218.

Johnston, M. (1994) Current Trends. *The Psychologist*, **7**(3), 114–118.

Kanner, A. D., Coyne, J. C., Schaeffer, C. and Lazarus, R. S. (1981) Comparison of two modes of stress measurement: Daily hassles and uplifts versus major life events. *Journal of Behavioural Medicine*, **4**, 1–39.

Kiecolt-Glaser, J. K., Glaser, R., Strain, E. C., Stout, J. C., Tarr, K. K., Holiday, J. E. and Speicher, C. E. (1986) Modulation of cellular immunity in medical students. *Journal of Behavioural Medicine*, **9**, 311–320.

Kulik, J. A. and Mahler, H. I. M. (1989) Social support and recovery from surgery. *Journal of Health Psychology* **8**, 221–238.

Lazarus, R. S. and Folkman, S. (1984) *Stress Appraisal and Coping*. Guildford, New York.

Lazarus, R. S., Kanner, A., and Folkman, S. (1980) *Emotions: A Cognitive-Phenomenological Analysis*. Academic Press, New York.

Lefcourt, H. M., Davidson-Katz, K. and Kueneman, K. (1990) Humour and immune system functioning. *Humour*, **3**, 305–321.

McEwen, B. S. and Stellar, E. (1998) Stress and the individual: Mechanisms leading to disease. *Archives of Internal Medicine*, 153, 2093–2101.

Meichenbaum, D. (1977) *Cognitive-Behaviour Modification: An Integrative Approach*. Plenum Press, New York.

Payne, R. and Firth-Cozens, J. (1987) *Stress in Health Professionals*. Wiley, New York.

Quine, L. (1998) Effects of stress in an NHS trust: A study. *Nursing Standard*, **13**,(3) 36–41.

Ragland, D. R. and Brand, R. J. (1988) Type A behaviour and mortality from coronary heart disease. *New England Journal of Medicine*, **318**, 65–69.

Schwartzner, R. and Leppin, A. (1992) *Social Support and Mental Health: A Conceptual and Empirical Overview*. Cited in Montada, L., Filipp, S. H. and Lerner, M. J. (eds) *Life Crises and Experience of Loss in Adult Life*. Erlbaum, Hillsdale, NJ.

Selye, H. (1956) *The Stress of Life*. McGraw-Hill, New York.

Selye, H. (1976) *Stress in Health and Disease*. Butterworth, Reading, MA.

Shouksmith, G. and Taylor, J. E. (1997) The interaction of culture with general job stressors in air traffic controllers. *International Journal of Aviation Psychology*, **7**, 343–352.

Spector, P. (2000) Employee control and occupational stress. *Current Directions in Psychological Science*, **11**, 133–136.

Wallis, B. and Fisher, L. E. (1987) *Consciousness and Behaviour*, 2nd edn. Allyn and Bacon, Boston.

Williams, R. B., Barefoot, J. C., Califf, R. M., Haney, T. L., Saunders, W. B., Pryor, D. B., Hlatky, M. A., Siegler, I. C. and Mark, D. B. (1992) Prognostic importance of social and economic resources among medically treated patients with angiographically documented coronary artery disease. *Journal of the American Medical Association*, **267**, 520–524.

Wills, T. A. (1984) *Supportive Functions of Interpersonal Relationships*. Cited in Cohen, S. and Syme, L., *Social Support and Health*. Academic Press, New York.

Chapter 10

Diseases and disorders

National unit specification
These are the topics you will be studying for this unit.

1   Historical developments in the field of biomedical science

2   Categories of disease

3   Epidemiological and experimental evidence of disease and disorders

4   The twenty-first century

1 Historical developments in the field of biomedical science

In industrialised society it is possible to use modern technology to extend and prolong human life far beyond the life span of those who lived in bygone eras. The patterns of infectious disease and mortality rates altered greatly during the twentieth century due to the development of effective drugs, surgical techniques, life-support systems and high standards of living.

Changing patterns of health are due to biological factors, and knowledge of disease and society's perception or definition of health also influence changes. The changes that occur in health and healthcare are due to political, structural, behavioural, cultural and technological changes that occur within society. In 1984 the World Health Organization (WHO) identified health as a multi-dimensional and shifting concept which cannot be easily analysed or measured. Healthcare workers must therefore be aware of the problems and dilemmas that may occur due to changes and advancements in healthcare.

Historical developments in the field of biomedical science have changed patterns of health and healthcare over the centuries.

Prehistoric man and ancient Egypt

Early civilisations based their beliefs on myths and legends. Humans are the only species known to man that are able to acknowledge that they will die, and this has influenced religious practice. Although the ancient civilisations acquired knowledge of anatomy, they were unable to comprehend the complexities of the human body. Disease was thought to be caused by spiritual beings, and healing was based on ridding the body of evil spirits. Evidence from 2600 BC shows that an Egyptian physician named Imphotep was worshipped as the god of healing.

The people of ancient Egypt had physicians and doctors to tend to the sick. Hieroglyphs found at the tomb of Irj dated 1500 BC describe him as a physician at the court of the pharaohs:

> 'Palace doctor, superintendent of the court physicians, palace eye physician, physician of the belly and one who understands the internal fluids and who is guardian of the anus'

Evidence of knowledge of anatomy is found through the inscriptions of the papyrus Ebers (1550 BC). The hieroglyphs describe the heart, pulse rates, blood, diet, massage, fasts, in addition to 700 medications used by Egyptian physicians.

Ancient Greece

The ancient Greek civilisations were the founders of medical science. Health was included as part of religious worship and the shrines to the gods emphasised the overall well-being of society. Temples were built to allow people to act out spiritual and social aspects of worship, and sports stadiums allowed athletes to offer their physical skills to the gods.

Hippocrates (460–375 BC) studied and developed a science of medicine that provided the foundations for the study of healthcare. His studies identified the relationship between internal harmony and the environment. Hippocrates was one of the great physicians of his time and his works include the Hippocratic Oath which has been used as the foundation of professional ethics.

The Hippocratic Oath

I swear by Apollo the healer, by Aesculapius, by Health and all the powers of healing, and call witness all the gods and goddesses that I may keep this Oath and Promise to the best of my ability and judgement.

I will pay the same respect to my master in the Science as to my parents and share my life with him and pay all my debts to him. I will regard his sons as my brothers and teach them the Science, if they desire to learn it, without fee or contract. I will hand on precepts, lectures and all other learning to my sons, to those of my master and to those pupils duly apprenticed and sworn, and to none other.

I will use my power to help the sick to the best of my ability and judgement; I will abstain from harming or wronging any man by it.

I will not give a fatal draught to anyone if I am asked, nor will I suggest any such thing. Neither will I give a woman means to procure an abortion.

I will be chaste and religious in my life and in my practice. I will not cut, even for the stone, but I will leave such procedures to the practitioners of that craft.

Whenever I go into a house, I will go to help the sick and never with the intention of doing harm or injury. I will not abuse my position to indulge in sexual contacts with the bodies of men or women, whether they be freemen or slaves.

Whatever I see or hear, professionally or privately, which ought not to be divulged, I will keep secret and tell no one.

If, therefore, I observe this Oath and do not violate it, may I prosper both in my life and in my profession, earning good repute among all men for all time. If I transgress and forswear this Oath, may my lot be otherwise.

The science of anatomy was developed by Galen (AD 130–200), a Greek physician. Although the use of human cadavers was forbidden, as a result of dissection work carried out on pigs and apes Galen was able to describe the structure of the brain and the cranial nerves, and suggest a theory for heartbeat. He was the first physician to use the pulse as a diagnostic aid. Galen continued the work of Hippocrates in his teachings on the relevance of observation and ideas concerning health and illness, and accumulated all known medical knowledge in a treatise that was used by physicians until the end of the middle ages.

Renaissance Europe

For many centuries the Christian Church dominated healthcare. Religious orders were established to care for the sick and needy. Men and women who practised healing were highly respected and valued members of society. During this period of time Europe suffered from outbreaks of the plague, cholera, typhoid and many other infectious diseases. Death was seen as God's will and it was not until the Renaissance period that medical science was allowed to progress beyond the confinement of religious doctrine. In AD 1000 a five-volume book of Greek and Arabic medicine was published, called the *Canon of Medicine*. The book, written by Avicenna, was used for reference by physicians until the seventeenth century.

In the eleventh century universities became established in Europe. Dissection of the human body, previously banned, was permitted, and the first book of anatomy, produced by Vesalius and entitled *On the Structure of the Human Body*, was published in 1543.

In 1560 Paracelsus, a physician who lived in Venice, expanded upon the works of Hippocrates. He believed that life could be prolonged by greater control over public health. To prove his theories, Paracelsus drained the swamp water away from Venice and reduced the pollution that was present in the Venetian harbour. Paracelsus also believed that personal health, including eating a healthy diet, was important for longevity. His work continued until he died aged 98.

The science of physiology was established in 1628 following the publication of the work of William Harvey. His work demonstrated the circulation of blood through the heart and vessels. This discovery was a major breakthrough leading the way for research of human physiology.

By the seventeenth century medical science was well established and this helped to bring about changes in healthcare. Although knowledge of anatomy, physiology and public health was accepted the general population continued to suffer from illness, disease and the effects of poverty. Herbal medicine was the only drug therapy available and surgical procedures were crude. Surgery on the battlefield was common and amputations were regularly performed in an attempt to prevent gangrene, but survival rates were low. Religious groups continued to look after the sick, providing care in hospitals and monasteries.

Advances in the eighteenth and nineteenth century

The eighteenth and nineteenth century saw the rapid development of medical knowledge. Scholars and physicians were able to use developing technology to assist them in discovering the secrets of the human body and the scientific links between health and disease.

Theories of respiration and gaseous exchange following experiments on gas analysis and the relationship between respiration and pulse rates were put forward by the chemist Antoine Lavoisier in 1794. His work was later used to continue studies in physiology, biochemistry and the concept of experimental medicine. In 1819 the first stethoscope was presented to the medical world as a diagnostic tool to allow physicians to hear changes that were occurring within the body.

Edward Jenner (1749–1823), an English country doctor, carried out observations and experiments that led to the first vaccination against smallpox. Jenner noticed that milkmaids sometimes milked cows that were suffering from cowpox. Those milkmaids, who consequently suffered from fever, inflammation and sores on their hands and wrists, never became ill with smallpox. In 1796 he took pus from the sores of a milkmaid with cowpox and transferred it to scratches he had made on the arms of a healthy boy. The boy went on to develop cowpox. When the boy recovered, Jenner repeated the experiment only this time he used pus from the sores of a person suffering from smallpox. The boy did not develop smallpox, thus supporting Jenner's theory. The experiment was repeated, and each time the person who had been infected with cowpox did not succumb to smallpox. The process of vaccinations proved to be very successful and this major development in healthcare was so effective that smallpox was later to be globally eradicated following a mass vaccination programme carried out by the World Health Organization.

In the seventeenth century Anton van Leeuwenhoek built a microscope and discovered the world of bacteria. The idea that disease was caused by a germ rather than evil spirits began the quest to identify the disease-causing organism. It was thought that bacteria appeared and generated spontaneously and although work continued on the germ theory of disease it was not until the middle of the nineteenth century that Louis Pasteur demonstrated the theory of contagion. Pasteur's work demonstrated the links between particular germs causing diseases such as anthrax, chicken pox and cholera. Using experiments based on the theory that microbes are found in the air, he successfully showed that the air in Paris contained far more microbes than were found in unpolluted mountain air. He discovered that some of the bacteria died when cultured with certain other bacteria, and this work lead to the first antibiotics being produced in 1939. His work included experiments to destroy the germs and he developed the process now known as pasteurisation. His original work was developed to prevent wine from turning sour, but the processes of heating fluid to 50–60° C also proved to be very successful in making milk safe for human consumption. His work on microbes also linked them to disease, and experiments using cholera and anthrax bacteria gave further evidence to support Jenner's work on vaccinations.

Pasteur had shown that it was possible to prevent and cure disease. His work, along with that of countless others, revolutionised healthcare and changed the pattern of health throughout Europe.

As society became more aware of the reasons for the illness and disease that blighted their lives, a greater awareness of personal health emerged. Public health was viewed as an area that required legislation to ensure control of water supplies, sanitation and food supplies.

The field of psychology was also gaining credibility following the work *New Theory of Vision* published in 1709 by George Berkley. William Wundt introduced experimental psychology in 1858. Wundt's theories were expanded upon by George John Romanes (comparative psychology) in 1883 and Sigmund Freud (psychoanalysis) in 1885.

In addition to knowledge being gained on the causes of disease, epoch-making events were also occurring in the field of surgery. Up until the nineteenth century surgery was a very traumatic and often fatal form of treatment. Surgeons were able to stop bleeding by tying ligatures around the bleeding vessels using thin strands of silk or catgut (catgut was obtained from the intestines of cows), cautery (using hot metal) or melted tar. These methods certainly did not make life any easier for the patient who had to endure the pain of surgery. Patients had to be tied down to immobilise them for surgery before the surgeon proceeded to cut. A skilled surgeon could amputate a limb and tie off the main arteries in little more than 30 seconds. If the patient survived this horrific procedure, the chance of the wound then becoming infected was very high due to the lack of an aseptic environment during and after surgery. In 1797 Humphrey Davy began work on the use of nitrous oxide as an aid to surgery. This gas, also known as laughing gas, meant that the patient could be anaesthetised during an operation, allowing the surgeon more time to perform surgery. The first published surgical procedure to take place while the patient was anaesthetised occurred in Boston in the US in 1846. In 1842 ether was first used as an anaesthetic, but the first documented case was not until 1846. Anaesthesia was a major breakthrough in the field of surgery although the patients at that time had a very low mortality rate due to post-operative infections. Fortunately a new technique in surgical procedures was being researched by the surgeon, Joseph Lister. He incorporated Pasteur's ideas on microorganisms and experimented by using carbolic acid as a disinfectant during surgery. The results dramatically reduced death rates following surgery and the use of antiseptic and aseptic techniques have been employed since. Surgical procedures developed rapidly within a relatively short period of time and in 1893 the first open heart surgery was performed by an American surgeon, Daniel Williams (Barnes-Svarney, 1995).

Twentieth-century medicine and healthcare

At the beginning of the twentieth century pioneering work in medicine and healthcare continued to develop at an incredible rate. Although social policies and healthcare began to improve, the quality of life for many people remained poor and life expectancy was short. Infectious diseases such as tuberculosis, scarlet fever, whooping cough, diphtheria, measles, typhoid and poliomyelitis thrived and one in seven children would not live past their seventh birthday. Childbirth carried a high maternal mortality rate and puerperal sepsis was common.

Although healthcare was available, it was often reserved for the wealthy. If the poorer members of society became ill, often the only option they had was the workhouse. The workhouse, founded on principles of charity, was regarded as a pauper's hospital. Conditions were harsh and regimes rigid. Often looked upon as an institute for the lowest echelons of society, the workhouse at least offered food and shelter. The industrial revolution had produced large areas of urbanisation and social problems of overcrowding, slum housing, inadequate sanitation and water supplies, and poor diet were common. Environmental pollution created by industrial machinery and processes added to the poor living conditions of the urban working class who lived in cramped and unhealthy homes. Working conditions were harsh and child labour was common. Life expectancy was short, and workers rarely lived beyond 30 years of age. Public health laws, food laws, employment laws and housing laws were introduced to raise the standards of living and reduce mortality rates.

Expectation of life at birth

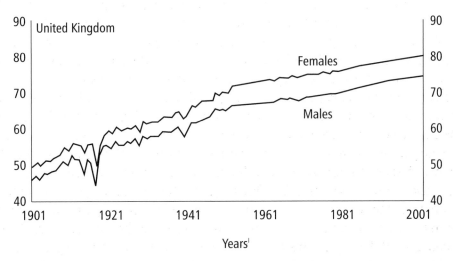

Years[1]

[1]Years indicates the number of years a new-born baby could be expected to live.

The development of therapeutic drugs made a huge impact on the health of society. Aspirin was the first synthetic drug, produced in 1899. This led on to the production of a wide array of drugs that effectively changed patterns of disease. Vaccinations and antibiotics reduced mortality rates dramatically and the introduction of diagnostic procedures including radiotherapy and biochemistry signalled the beginning of an era where prevention and treatment of illness changed perceptions and patterns of health throughout industrialised society.

The twentieth century

During the twentieth century scientists were able to study disease and disorders in far greater depth than ever before due to the amazing advances made in the field of technology. The list of achievements made in the field of healthcare is vast, from diagnostic procedures through to treatment and prevention of disease and disorders. Radiotherapy, psychiatry, biochemistry, electronic engineering, physics, physiology, polymer science, psychology, surgery, immunology and genetic engineering are a few of the diverse sciences that have contributed to the advances in medicine and healthcare.

The twentieth century saw the eradication of various diseases and, for many, an improvement in living conditions and lifestyle. Life span increased to the extent that there were new healthcare demands to care for an increasing number of elderly people. New diseases emerged that were the result of affluent lifestyles, and circulatory disease became the biggest threat to health.

Despite all of the advances made, the poor still remained the most vulnerable and susceptible to illness and disease. Finance for new technology led to many ethical debates on who should and should not have treatment. The question of finance remains unresolved.

2 Categories of disease

A major advancement made in the twentieth century was the classification of disease. Disease is a broad term that is used to describe an illness or disorder causing physical or psychological disturbance to homeostasis in the human body. The study of disease and the disease processes is called pathology.

Disease or disorder may be caused by a single factor or it may be multifactorial. In pathology most disease can be placed into a broad type or category.

Birth defects

- Inherited: a genetic abnormality that has been inherited from one or both parents at the time of fertilisation of the egg.

- Congenital: an abnormality present from birth. The disease or disorder is caused by teratogens. Teratogen is the collective name for environmental factors that cause physical problems that are present at birth. There is no genetic link and the disease or disorder is acquired *in utero*.

Acquired

- Injury: injury to body tissue by a physical cause, e.g. trauma, heat, cold, irradiation and chemicals.

- Inflammations: this group includes all infections due to bacteria, viruses, parasites, worms and fungi.

- Mechanical: diseases that result from mechanical failure within the body, e.g. intestinal obstruction.

- Metabolic: all diseases that cause metabolic disturbances due to starvation or deprivation of specific nutritional substances. This includes vitamin deficiencies as well as diseases such as gout, which is due to an intrinsic metabolic abnormality.

- Circulatory: this group of diseases encompasses all disorders of the heart, blood vessels and blood together with the abnormalities of circulation, e.g. oedema and thrombosis.

- Endocrine: diseases caused by abnormal function of the endocrine glands.

- Degenerations and infiltrations: all disease processes that cause retrogressive changes in the body cells.

- Tumours: benign or malignant tumours.

- Other varieties: any disease of an unknown nature or which is idiopathic. This includes disease of a psychiatric origin.

Pathology uses the medical model of health to study disease. Clinical specialities within the field of medicine are often based on the categories used in pathology, for example a trauma specialist or a cancer specialist. Modern technology and research widened knowledge of disease and disorders showing that although one single factor may cause a disease, the results may well have a multifactorial effect. Likewise disease and disorders often have predisposing causes that may be due to physical, psychological or social factors.

The introduction of the biopsychosocial model of health required new categories of disease to be created that would allow for the multifactorial cause and effect of disease. The following categories of disease and disorders allow healthcare workers to view care as a holistic concept ensuring that all multifactorial aspects are included when planning and implementing care.

Categories of disease and disorders

Category	Cause of disease	Example
Physical	Temporary or permanent damage to any part of the body. Includes all other categories except mental that has no physical cause	Trauma
Infectious	Organisms that invade the body	HIV Malaria
Non-infectious	Any cause other than invading organism	Cancer
Degenerative Deficiency	Gradual decline in function Poor diet	Osteoporosis Scurvy
Inherited or congenital	A genetic fault inherited from one or both parents Congenital defect present at birth	Tay-Sachs disease Cystic fibrosis
Mental	Changes to the mind due to physical cause or unknown	Manic depression
Social	Social behaviour and environment	Drug dependency Malnutrition
Self-inflicted	Damage caused to the body by a person's own action	Lung cancer Attempted suicide

Although the table places disease into different categories, disease or effects of the disease may belong to more than one category. In a social disease such as drug dependency the overriding problem may be classed as social but the effects will lead to problems in all other categories, for example:

- Physical: damage to arteries and skin due to injections of drugs; damage to nasal septum if inhaling drugs.

- Infectious: septic sores at injection site; HIV; hepatitis.

- Non-infectious: ulcer.

- Deficiency: vitamin deficiencies due to poor diet.

- Degenerative: dementia – due to treatable cause.

- Mental: drug-induced psychosis.

- Self-inflicted: lung cancer if drugs inhaled via smoking.

Acute and chronic disease

Disease may be classed as acute or chronic. Acute disease has a sudden onset causing rapid changes that last for a short period of time. The signs and symptoms of an acute illness appear very quickly and the disease is self-limiting. A common cold is classed as an acute disease and a full recovery is usually made after the disease has run its course. Acute meningitis has a very rapid onset, but recovery is uncertain as this disease carries a high mortality rate. In both cases the disease is self-limiting.

Chronic disease often has a insidious beginning with slow progression of the disease. The effects of a chronic illness may last for months or years. An acute illness that continues to disrupt homeostasis may progress to a chronic illness. There may also be acute periods during chronic illness. Chronic illness often has debilitating effects that affect a person's quality of life, for example chronic obstructive airways disease limits physical activity due to a shortness of breath following minimal exertion.

Physical diseases

This category of disease incorporates all physical damage caused by disease itself or damage to tissue cells caused by the disruption in homeostasis. Injury and trauma are obvious causes of physical disease, but all categories of disease will have an impact on the anatomy and physiology of the body. In 1997, 42 967 people were seriously injured and 280 978 slightly injured in road traffic accidents, about 800 000 people were injured while playing sport, and accidents in the home (including falls, burns, poisoning, cuts and choking) accounted for one-third of all accidents (*Saving Lives: Our Healthier Nation*, Government White Paper, 1999). Infectious disease such as polio may produce long-term effects on the body, causing varying degrees of paralysis, while a social disease such as alcoholism may lead to a wide variety of physical diseases including liver damage and pancreatitis.

Infectious diseases

Organisms that live in or on the human body and gain nutrition from the host body are called parasites. Ectoparasites live on the skin while endoparasites are internal. If the parasites cause disease they are described as pathogens.

Infectious or communicable diseases are caused by pathogens being transmitted from one host to another. The host may be a human or an animal. Pathogens that affect the human body include:

- Viruses, e.g. chicken pox, herpes zoster, mumps, measles, HIV.

A virus

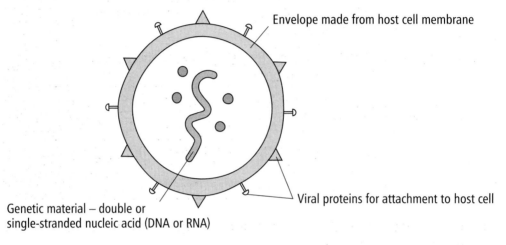

Envelope made from host cell membrane

Viral proteins for attachment to host cell

Genetic material – double or single-stranded nucleic acid (DNA or RNA)

The HIV virus uses its genetic material to make more copies of itself inside human cells. There are one million nanometres (nm) in a millimetre and viruses range in size from 10 nm to 300 nm.

- Bacteria, e.g. tetanus, botulism, anthrax.

Bacterium – general structure

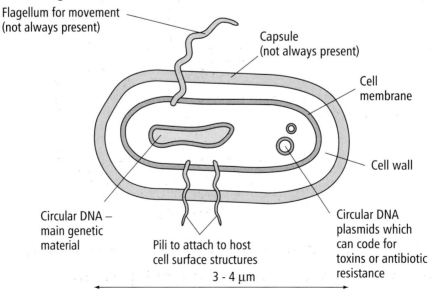

Flagellum for movement (not always present)

Capsule (not always present)

Cell membrane

Cell wall

Circular DNA – main genetic material

Pili to attach to host cell surface structures

Circular DNA plasmids which can code for toxins or antibiotic resistance

3 - 4 µm

Bacteria are spherical or rod-shaped structures that are the smallest organism to have a cellular structure. There are many forms of bacteria and in the right environment binary fusion will occur every 20 minutes causing rapid growth of a bacterial colony.

Bacteria under a microscope

Shape	Example	Disease caused	Shape	Example	Disease caused
Spherical (cocci) Single			Rod-shaped (baccilli) Single	Escherichia coli	Gastroenteritis
Chains	Streptococcus pyrogens	Scarlet fever	Chains	Bacillus anthracis	Anthrax
Clumps	Staphylococcus aureus	Boils Pneumonia	Flagellate	Salmonella typhi	Typhoid fever
Pairs in a capsule	Diplococcus pneumoniae	Pneumonia	Spiral-shaped (spirillum)	Treponemia pallidum	Syphilis
Pairs	Neisseria gonorrhoea	Gonorrhoea	Comma-shaped (vibro)	Vibrio cholerae	Cholera

Bacteria are large enough to be seen under a light microscope and different forms of bacteria cause specific diseases.

- Fungi, e.g. candida albicans (thrush), athlete's foot.

Fungus

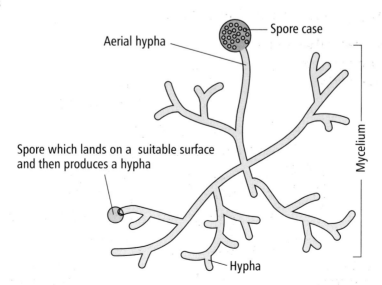

Fungi cannot make their own food and they feed on living or dead organisms.

- Protozoa, e.g. malaria, trypanosomiasis (sleeping sickness).

Protozoa

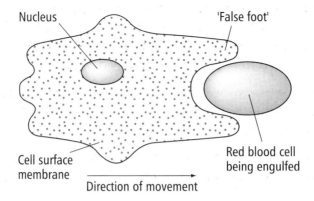

Protozoa are one-celled parasitic organisms. This protozoa is called Entamoeba and it causes dysentery.

- Worms, e.g. round worm, tapeworms, flukes.

Worms

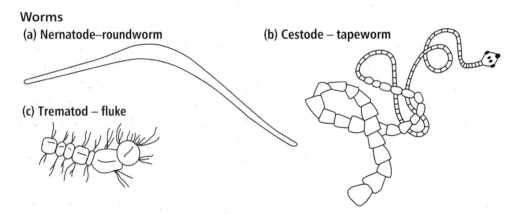

(a) Nernatode–roundworm

(b) Cestode – tapeworm

(c) Trematod – fluke

The most common round-worm disease in the UK is threadworm infestation. Tapeworms are usually acquired by eating undercooked meat or fish. Two main diseases caused by flukes are liver fluke and schistosomiasis (a tropical disease).

- Insect, e.g. head louse, scabies.

Insect

(a) Mite

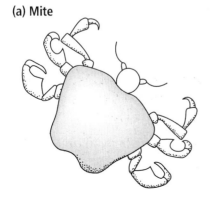

(b) Pediculus humanus capitis – head louse

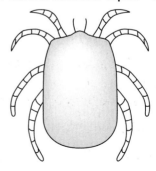

The mite *Sarcoptes scabiei* burrows into the skin to lay eggs. Scabies infestations cause intense itching and are highly contagious, being transmitted by close physical contact. A louse is a wingless insect that feeds on human blood. *Pediculus humanus capitis* (head louse), *pediculus humanus corporis* (body louse) and *phthirus pubis* (pubic louse/crab) are spread by direct contact.

Infectious disease may be transmitted in a number of ways including social or physical contact with an infected person, contaminated water or food, airborne infection, droplet infection or animal vectors.

In some infectious diseases the host becomes a carrier of the pathogen. The carrier does not have the symptoms of the disease but they transmit the pathogen to others.

Infectious diseases are the leading cause of global mortality and debility and account for approximately one-third of all deaths and more than two-thirds of child deaths. Infectious diseases and malnutrition are largely responsible for the difference in infant mortality rates and life expectancies between developed and developing countries (United Nations, 1989).

The development of vaccines and immunisation programmes are useful in eradicating, eliminating and controlling infectious disease that causes widescale illness within society. For vaccinations to be effective in preventing epidemics of disease, the majority of the population must be immunised. The use of vaccines is beneficial to protect individuals against disease and it is a cost-effective method of preventative medicine. The disadvantages of mass immunisation include possible allergic reaction to live vaccines, extreme immune responses and a possible link to the rise in childhood asthma and allergies.

Chemical control of infectious diseases using antimicrobial or antiviral drugs (in particular antibiotics) is used to interfere with the metabolism of the microorganism whilst causing minimal damage to the body tissues. Over-usage of antibiotics has caused mutated, drug-resistant strains of bacteria, creating the commonly named 'superbugs'.

A localised incidence of infectious disease is called an outbreak; a national increase is called an epidemic. An endemic disease is one that is common in a particular population all of the time. An endemic disease that affects different countries at the same time is called a pandemic.

Non-infectious diseases

If a disease has no known pathogen it will be called a non-infectious disease. The disease may be due to one or more disorders and may affect any organ or tissue within the body. Examples of non-infectious disease are:

- Anaemia.

- Dermatitis.

- Cerebrovascular incident (stroke).

- Psoriasis.

- Raynaud's disease.

- Irritable bowel syndrome.

- Haemorrhoids.

- Varicose veins.

- Headaches.

Non-infectious disease may be caused by trauma, environment, inherited disorder, lifestyles or deficiency diseases.

Deficiency diseases

Humans require a supply of organic food to provide the nutrients necessary for growth, repair and energy. Diet must contain proteins, lipids, carbohydrates, inorganic ions, vitamins, dietary fibre and water. The diet must be balanced to provide the correct amounts of nutritional substances to maintain homeostasis. An inadequate or unbalanced intake will lead to deficiency diseases.

Deficiency diseases are often chronic disorders and may be due to:

- An inadequate dietary intake – poor diet, social (i.e. due to finance, lifestyle, religion, depression, anorexia nervosa etc.).

- Gastrointestinal malabsorption – this occurs when the body is unable to digest the nutrients. The most common causes in the UK are coeliac disease, Crohn's disease and chronic pancreatitis. Infections, bacteria and defective secretions of gastric juices may also lead to symptoms of deficiencies. Deficiency disease may present as a post-operative complication following surgery of the gastrointestinal tract.

Malnutrition may be due to starvation or self-imposed eating habits. In industrialised nations slimming diets are sometimes a cause of dietary deficiency diseases.

Diseases are also caused by intolerance to food, for example lactose intolerance and food allergies.

Inherited diseases

Congenital disorders

In many cases congenital disorders are the result of social and infectious diseases and are therefore not true inherited disease. However, the majority of disorders have no known cause and may be classified depending on the disease, i.e. physical and non-infectious. An example of congenital disease is Fetal Alcohol Syndrome (FAS) caused by the mother drinking alcohol during pregnancy. FAS babies are born prematurely, have facial abnormalities and may suffer deformities of major internal organs including the brain. As they develop, many will suffer from dental, auditory, visual and spinal disorders. Intellectual and psychological impairment persist throughout their lives.

Inherited disease

Geneticists have recognised that genes are located on rod-shaped structures called chromosomes in the body's cells. Chromosomes are usually found in pairs, except for two chromosomes found in males. The genes appear in the same order and place along the chromosome. The different forms for a particular gene, for example eye or hair colour, are called alleles.

The exact number of different genes in the human body is unknown, but there are probably about 100,000 functional genes. Genes determine the traits that are inherited from parents and they control the activities that take place in our cells throughout our lifetime. Genetic defects may be caused by changes in the nitrogenous base sequence of the gene which result in a faulty allele or version of the gene. The mutation produced may lead to a number of inherited diseases including predisposition (i.e. a special tendency) to illness if environmental triggers are encountered. The faulty allele may be found on one or both genes and inherited diseases are often categorised on the inheritance pattern.

Examples of inherited disease are as follows.

Diseases due to dominant inheritance:

- Achondroplasia.
- Huntingdon's chorea.
- Multiple neurofibromatosis.

Diseases due to recessive inheritance:

- Phenylketonuria.
- Cystic fibrosis.

Diseases due to X-linked recessive inheritance:

- Muscular dystrophy.
- Haemophilia.
- Colour blindness.

Sex limited traits:

- Baldness.

Multifactorial inheritance:

- Hare lip.

- Congenital dislocation of the hip.

Inherited diseases may be present at birth or develop in later life. A familiar disease is one that occurs within a family group or 'runs in the family', for example breast cancer, bowel cancer and coronary heart disease. The mutated gene may need to respond to an environmental trigger before the disease develops.

There was no cure for inherited diseases in the past, but recent advances in the knowledge of genetics has enabled geneticists to correct or replace the faulty allele in diseases that affect the immune system using a technique called gene therapy. Sufferers of cystic fibrous have had some symptoms of their disease alleviated by the use of a nasal spray that has been developed using genetic engineering.

Diagnostic tests for several inherited diseases are available using DNA extracted from blood or cheek scrapings. The tests can identify whether a person is a carrier of a faulty allele and this test is often used as an antenatal genetic test for cystic fibrosis, sickle-cell anaemia and thalassaemia. Screening tests are also offered to clients who may be at risk from alzheimer's disease, breast cancer and ovarian cancer.

If requested, a fetus may be checked for genetic abnormalities early in pregnancy using techniques including chorionic villi sampling, amniocentesis and ultrasound imaging (Stranc *et al.*, 1997).

Genetic research has offered hope to sufferers of inherited disease and it may be possible to greatly reduce the number of inherited diseases in the future. However, genetic research does raise a number of ethical issues that need to be addressed, including the ownership of identified genetic codes. (If a company has found a genetic code, do they keep the code a company secret and use the information to produce profit-making 'cures'?)

Degenerative diseases

The genetic codes in the human body act as a genetic clock that triggers a process of physiological decline in adults called ageing.

Degenerative diseases may occur at any age but they are more commonly associated with the process of ageing.

Degenerative diseases are amongst those being treated by tissue engineering. This research is still in the early stages of development and involves new tissue being grown in laboratories to replace damaged tissue. At the present time, laboratory-grown versions of skin and cartilage are available, but work continues on producing bone, tendons, heart valves, bone marrow, brain cells, intestines, liver and kidneys.

There are three main types of degenerative disease:

- Diseases of the nervous system, skeletal system and muscular system.
- Diseases of the cardiovascular system.
- Cancer.

Diseases of the nervous, skeletal and muscular system

Nerves

Degenerative diseases of the nervous system may be caused by disorders of the myelin sheath and synaptic dysfunction.

Deterioration of the myelin sheath

An example of this is multiple sclerosis (MS), an autoimmune disease that causes a progressive destruction of the myelin sheath. It occurs more in women than men and usually appears between the age of 20 and 40 years. The body's own immune system attacks the myelin sheath causing sclerosis. Patches of sclerosis prevent conduction of nerve impulses. The most common form of MS has periods of remission and relapse. The cause of MS is not known but it may be linked to genetic susceptibility or viral infection.

Inflammatory demyelinating disease

Swelling, oedema and demyelination of nerves may occur due to infections, deficiencies, toxins, metabolic disorders and genetic disorders.

Synaptic dysfunction

If problems occur involving the secretion and synthesis of neurotransmitters, messages will not be able to travel along the nervous system. Examples of synaptic dysfunction are:

- Myasthenia gravis: in this condition there are not enough muscle acetyl-choline receptors which leads to muscle weakness. This disorder usually develops in early adulthood and may progress to permanent weakness.

- Parkinson's disease: this is due to the degeneration of dopamineric neu-rones in the substantia nigra. In the early stages of Parkinson's disease signs of loss of muscle control and cognitive function are displayed.

Skeletal tissue

Degenerative disease of the skeletal system is more pronounced in women than men during the ageing process. Women lose bone mass and calcium from the bones to a greater extent than men due to female hormonal changes following the menopause. This makes women more susceptible to osteoporosis. Degeneration of bone will also lead to bone brittleness, bone deformity, pain, stiffness and loss of teeth.

Reduction in bone mass may also be caused by excessive wear and tear (for example the hip joint), deficiency disease due to low calcium intake, hereditary disease such as brittle bone syndrome, cancer or environmental factors.

Muscle

Skeletal muscle degenerates with progressive loss of muscle mass from the age of about 30 years. The muscle mass is replaced by fibrous connective and adipose tissue. The muscle reflexes become slower and there will be a decrease in strength.

If muscle fibres are not used regularly, wasting will occur. This is called muscular atrophy. Degeneration of myofibrils and nerves is common in clients who are bedridden or have spinal cord injuries.

Diseases of the cardiovascular system

Degenerative disease of the cardiovascular system is often a common problem associated with ageing. The signs and symptoms of degenerative disease include:

- Atherosclerosis.
- Hardening of the aorta.
- Reduction in muscle fibre of the cardiac muscle.
- Weakening of cardiac muscle strength.
- Reduced cardiac output.
- Lower heart rate.
- Increase in systolic blood pressure.

Degeneration of the tissues occurs in ageing due to an imbalance of glucose affecting protein molecules. Cross-links between protein molecules are formed which causes stiffening and loss of elasticity in tissue. Elastin within the blood vessels thickens and calcium is deposited leading to the possible development of atherosclerosis.

Diseases of the cardiovascular system account for over 200,000 deaths in the UK each year, with England having the highest rate of coronary heart disease in western Europe (WHO, 1995).

The causes of cardiovascular disease are linked to lifestyle and genetic traits.

Cancer

Cancer is the termed used to describe a group of diseases that produce an uncontrolled division of abnormal cells. The cells develop into a mass called a tumour. A malignant tumour is a destructive growth that is able to metastasise (spread) to other organs. The cancerous cells invade body tissue, taking the nutrients and growing in size, causing degeneration of normal tissue. There are different types of cancer depending upon the type of tissue affected:

- Carcinomas (kar'-si-NŌ-maz): cancer that originates from epithelial cells.

- Melanomas (mel'-a-NŌ-maz): cancer that originates in melanocytes (skin cancer).

- Sarcoma (sar-KŌ-ma): cancer that originates in muscle or connective tissue (includes bone cancer).

- Leukaemia (loo-KĒ-mē-a): abnormal leukocytes causing cancer of the blood.

Cancer may be caused as a result of environmental triggers or carcinogens or as a result of abnormal genes. Treatment of cancer includes surgery, chemotherapy, radiation and immunotherapy.

Mental disorders

If a disease or illness affects a person's behaviour, emotions, thoughts, memory or social behaviour it is classed as a mental disorder. Mental disorder may be caused by a physical, infective, non-infective, degenerative, inherited, deficiency or self-inflicted disorder or have no obvious cause. Neurological studies continue to develop new ideas and rationale of the cause of as yet unknown factors that cause mental disorders.

Physical signs of mental disorders are associated with abnormal physiology, degeneration of brain tissue, or as the result of physical trauma. In many incidences of mental disease changes in the patterns of blood flow or imbalances in the secretion of neurotransmitters in the brain may be observed.

Infectious diseases such as Creutzfeldt-Jakob disease (CJD) cause large areas of brain tissue to be destroyed resulting in loss of mental faculties and coordination. Brain damage is severe and this disease is fatal.

Progressive degeneration of the brain cells due to a decreased production in acetylcholine is a sign of Alzheimer's. This disease is more common in people over the age of 65 years, but it may begin at any age. The cause is unknown but there is an increased familial incidence that suggests a possible genetic link. The onset is insidious with the slow deterioration of all mental faculties causing acute confusion.

Mental disorders vary in the degree of severity, and treatment will depend on the cause.

Mental disorders are usually classified using the International Classification of Disease (ICD) that was developed by the World Health Organization. The American Psychiatric Association use the ICD categories of disorders in their *Diagnostic and Statistical Manual of Mental Disorders* (*DSM*) which is recognised internationally as a guide to diagnosis (Field, 2003).

The fourth edition of the *DSM* was revised in 1994 and the following categories are based on diagnostic criteria of mental disorders excluding personality disorders and mental retardation:

- Disorders first diagnosed in infancy, childhood or adolescence that include behavioural problems and problems with cognitive and social development.

- Delirium, dementia, amnesia and other cognitive disorders caused by physical or degenerative disease.

- Substance-related disorders leading to psychological distress.

- Schizophrenia and other psychotic disorders that are characterised by a detachment from reality and severe emotional and social disturbances.

- Mood disorders including depression.

- Anxiety disorders including panic attacks, phobias and obsessive compulsive disorder.

- Somatoform disorders.

- Dissociative disorders where a person has an alternative or multiple identities.

- Sexual and gender identity disorders including physical disorders of sexual performance such as premature ejaculation and paraphilias (the name given to disorders in which sexual pleasure is gained using antisocial acts such as necrophilia, paedophilia and exhibitionism).

- Eating disorders including anorexia nervosa and bulimia nervosa.

- Sleeping disorders including insomnia and sleepwalking.

- Impulse control disorders including pyromania and obsessive gambling.

- Adjustment disorders, being unable to cope with a stressful event.

The complex interrelationship between the mind and body often makes it difficult to differentiate mental and physical ill health and it is therefore important to provide a holistic approach to diagnosis and care.

Social diseases

Patterns of illness and disease have changed over the last century and although cures and prevention of disease is now affective against infectious disease, new illnesses that are connected to our social environment have become just as fatal. The present government White Paper, *Saving Lives: Our Healthier Nation*, states that the social, economic and environmental factors tending towards poor health are considerable (1999). The Black Report (1980) showed evidence that people who lived in low social-economic groups suffered from increased rates of nearly all categories of disease that affected them throughout their lives.

Social conditions that affect health are numerous. The main factors creating increased incidence of social disease are as follows.

Income

The lifestyle that people adopt is often based on their income. Those on a high income are able to afford housing, warmth, a healthy diet, private transport and leisure activities. Success is usually achieved through work and self-belief often related to education and degree of qualifications and skills. Those on a lower income or those on social security benefits are more likely to die younger from diseases such as cancer, cardiovascular disease and accidents (Harding *et al.*, 1999).

Housing

The type of housing in which people live has an impact on health. If housing is overcrowded, damp, cold, with poor lighting, no recreational area and with an increased accident risk and/or fire potential, the impact on health will be negative. Cold and damp conditions aggravate respiratory disease and other medical conditions including asthma, bronchitis, rheumatism and arthritis. Overcrowding increases the incidence of infectious diseases (i.e. tuberculosis and dysentery), the spread of infection, insomnia and stress. Accident rates, especially amongst children, are higher in areas of overcrowding. The high-rise tower blocks and estates built in the 1950s and 1960s saw an increase in mental illness, especially depression, and low self-esteem due to the social isolation created by the architectural design. Control of rodents (rats and mice) and insects (cockroaches, fleas, lice etc.) is more difficult in urban areas, especially areas of substandard housing.

Diet

A person's diet has a marked influence on health. Deficiency disease affects homeostasis, and diets high in salt, sugar and fatty foods and low in fibre are linked to cardiovascular disease, cancers of the bowel and tooth decay. Income and lifestyle have a major impact on diet. In industrialised countries there has been a huge increase in consumption of convenience foods containing high levels of salt, sugar and additives. This has in part been due to the changing structure of society.

Physical fitness and recreation

Levels of physical activity vary depending on income, occupation and social group. Physical inactivity is responsible for increased incidence of cardiovascular disease, obesity and osteoporosis. Obesity in itself may predispose illness including diabetes. In 1996 25% of women in the low socio-economic group aged 16 and over were found to be obese compared with 14% in the professional socio-economic group (Prescott-Clarke and Primatesta, 1998). Obesity is becoming an increasing healthcare problem in children and adults.

Environmental and occupational disease

Environmental and occupational diseases are those caused by harmful external environments.

Occupational disease

The health, safety and welfare of all workers in the UK is protected by the Health and Safety at Work Act 1974 and enforced by the Health and Safety Commission. In 1988 Control of Substances Hazardous to Health (COSHH) Regulations were set up to control the 100 000-plus chemicals in everyday use. Further regulations, including the Reporting of Injuries, Disease and Dangerous Occurrences Regulations 1985 (RIDDOR), have been introduced to control and maintain safe working environments and these also cover food hygiene. Occupational disease in healthcare includes back injuries, stress, infections (including methicillin-resistant staphylococcus aureus, HIV, hepatitis and influenza), and industrial injuries due to fire and faulty equipment. Infection control and safe working practices are extremely important areas of healthcare aimed at preventing the spread of avoidable disease.

Environmental disease

Environmental factors that increase the risk of disease include:

- Climate: hot, damp climates promote the growth of bacteria. Death from infectious and parasitic disease is far higher in developing countries (WHO, 1992).

- Geography: urban or rural area. Overcrowding in urban areas increases the risk of stress, infectious disease and pollution. Patterns of disease may relate to geographical location. For example, houses in Cornwall are often built over granite. Granite emits high levels of radon gas that predisposes lung cancer.

- Air pollution: damage to the ozone layer in the stratosphere has altered the proportions of natural gases in the air. The following pollutants are also air-borne:
    - Smoke: comprises of small particles of carbon that may affect the epithelial lining of the alveoli. It causes respiratory problems and bronchitis.
    - Sulphuric acid: released into the air when fossil fuel is burnt and during the smelting of ore. Extra mucous is produced by the goblet cells and cilia become dysfunctional and unable to remove the increased mucous containing trapped dirt and bacteria. Gaseous exchange is affected and the alveoli may be damaged. Bronchitis and respiratory tract infections are common.
    - Smog: smog occurs in areas where fog remains static. Pollutants from fossil-fuel fires become trapped in the fog causing smog.
    - Lead: petrol exhaust was found to be a major cause of lead pollution in the atmosphere. Lead poisoning causes abdominal pain, diarrhoea, vomiting, anaemia and damage to the nervous system. Acute poisoning may be fatal.

- Water pollution: natural water is rarely pure as it absorbs chemicals from the air and soil. High concentrations of additives resulting from human activities, such as industrial work, cause pollutants. Harmful pollutants include:
    - Untreated water supply may contain infectious diseases and poisons. Water-borne diseases include parasitic worms, protozoa, cholera, typhoid and poliomyelitis.
    - Sewage: untreated sewage contains potentially harmful bacteria.
    - Industrial pollutants: the waste chemicals used in industry may contaminate water directly or indirectly. Mercury (causing paralysis, convulsions, blindness and death), lead and aluminium (causing disease of the brain, liver, lungs and thyroid gland) are chemicals commonly found in industrial waste.

- Noise: unwanted sound or noise is considered to be a form of pollution. Constant noise may cause damage to hearing and, with very loud noise, rupture of the eardrums and damage to the ossicles is possible. Persistent low-intensity sounds affect psychological health by causing stress, tiredness and loss of concentration – leading to an increased risk of accidents.

Self-inflicted diseases

Personal behaviour and lifestyle may lead to disease. Decisions made about personal behaviour are usually made by individuals, but if the behaviour is a well-known risk to health any resulting disease will be classed as self-inflicted. Deliberate self harm, including attempted suicide, is regarded as a self-inflicted illness although the actual cause is often poor mental health. In industrialised countries suicide is a major cause of mortality in young people, particularly males (Aylin *et al.*, 1999).

Substance abuse

Lifestyle and behaviour will depend on socioeconomic groups and the structure of society. Substance abuse occurs when a person takes drugs that are harmful to health. This excludes taking drugs for medicinal reasons or moderate amounts of social drugs such as caffeine or alcohol.

At the beginning of the twentieth century, opium addiction was a recognised social disease and sanatoriums to treat drug habits were available for the wealthy. Inebriety due to the consumption of alcohol was a major problem. In September 1905 a report presented to parliament by the Medical Officer of Health concluded that 'alcoholism is the most terrible enemy to public health, to family happiness, and to national prosperity, and even to the future of the race' (Priestley, 1905). The problems identified in 1905 remain the same in 2004 as alcohol is still a socially acceptable drug.

Alcohol

Alcohol is a depressant and it reduces activity of the brain, affecting self-control, coordination and judgement. In the short term, alcohol abuse may lead to physical injury and it is estimated that up to 40 000 deaths per year could be alcohol related. Alcohol abuse is closely linked with violence, leading to increased problems of domestic abuse, child abuse, sexual offences, crime and physical assaults/murder. Long-term alcohol abuse increases the risk of:

- Alcohol dependency.
- Cirrhosis of the liver.
- Cancer of the mouth, throat, oesophagus and liver.
- Psychological and emotional disorders (violence, depression).
- Obesity.
- Deficiency disorders.
- Cerebral vascular incidence (strokes).

Smoking

The smoking of tobacco is a major cause of preventable disease in the western world. Smokers have a higher risk of disease and illness due to the harmful chemicals found in tobacco. Nicotine is one of the many chemicals found in tobacco. It is a powerful, fast-acting and highly addictive drug. The immediate effects of nicotine on homeostasis occur within minutes and cause:

- An increase in heart rate and blood pressure.
- Vasoconstriction.
- Changes in blood composition.
- Changes in appetite.

Health risks of cigarette smoking include:

- Bronchitis.
- Pneumonia.
- Emphysema.
- Stroke.
- Cancer of the mouth, throat and oesophagus.
- Cancer of the larynx.
- Coronary heart disease.
- Chronic obstructive pulmonary disease.
- Lung cancer.
- Pancreatic cancer.
- Ulcers.
- Bladder cancer.
- Peripheral vascular disease.
- Cervical cancer.
- Premature and low-birth weight babies.

Smoking-related disease is more prevalent in lower socio-economic groups and as indicated in the government White Paper *Smoking Kills* (1998) the reduction of tobacco smoking will have a huge impact on reducing mortality rates. Due to the highly addictive nature of tobacco it may not be easy to reduce the number of people who smoke. The use of nicotine therapy has proved successful in helping to reduce the side effects of withdrawal from smoking, but a greater number of people are now addicted to nicotine substitutes. By failing to treat the drug addiction there is an increased risk of returning to the smoking habit.

Drugs

Any drug will cause harm if it is not used correctly. Misuse of drugs is a growing problem in industrialised society particularly amongst the young.

Non-prescription illegal drugs are substances that are associated with short-term effects that produce feelings of pleasure, mental stimulation and physical energy. Taken over prolonged periods, psychological dependency, physiological side effects and social disorders may occur. Commonly misused medicinal and illegal drugs include the following.

Commonly misused medicinal and illegal drugs

Type of drug	Dangers
Amphetamines: stimulant that is sniffed, injected or swallowed. Very addictive	Disturbed sleep, loss of appetite, increased respiratory and heart rate, raised blood pressure, anxiety and/or paranoia
Anabolic steroids: increase muscle size, abused by some athletes and body builders	Stimulates aggression, causes jaundice and depression and affects reproductive hormones leading to infertility
Barbiturates: sedative **Cannabis:** relaxant	Physical and mental dependence Induces a false sense of well-being. It is often combined with tobacco and long-term use will increase the risk of smoking-related diseases
Cocaine: powerful stimulant made from the leaves of the Andean coca shrub. May be injected or inhaled to produce feelings of mental exhilaration, indifference to pain and illusions of physical and mental strength	Cocaine is highly addictive and induces dependence. It is expensive to buy. Patterns of behaviour may change and anti-social behaviour including theft and prostitution are common in order for the user to afford to buy the drug. Injections lead to vascular disorders and increased risk of blood-borne disease. Deficiency disorders and increased risk of sexually transmitted disease are common. Anxiety and panic attacks are a side-effect of the drug. Overuse may lead to respiratory distress
Ecstasy (methylenedioxymethamphetamine): synthetic drug with hypnotic properties used to heighten perception	Repeated use carries a risk of liver damage. The most common side-effect is hyperthermia leading to intense thirst and consumption of excessive fluids. Oedema will follow, leading to heart and kidney failure and swelling of brain tissue. Distorted vision with altered perceptions of self.
LSD (d-lysergic acid diethylamide): hallucinogenic drug	Side-effects include depression, dizziness and panic attacks
Magic mushrooms: a type of mushroom that grows wild in the UK. It contains psilocybin which is classed as a hypnotic drug Solvents (aerosol sprays, butane gas, solvent-based glue, paint, dry-cleaning fluid, correction fluids petrol etc.)	The hypnotic effects may lead to over-excitement and hallucinations. Side effects include vomiting and severe abdominal pain Solvent abuse is popular amongst some teenagers as the toxic substances are cheap and easy to obtain. Dangers from substance abuse include inhalation of vomit, suffocation due to oedema and drowning due to disorientation and feelings of recklessness. Long-term abuse increases the risk of disease of bone marrow, liver, kidneys, respiratory and nervous system

The use of recreational drugs has been observed in many societies throughout the ages and, as in the past, debate continues about personal liberty and freedom versus social responsibility.

Drug misuse is associated with poor health and social exclusion through homelessness, poverty, unemployment and criminal behaviour (*Saving Lives: Our Healthier Nation*, Government White Paper 1999).

Sexually transmitted disease (STD)

Sexual activity involves personal risk and exposure to sexually transmitted disease. The most common diseases in men and women are chlamydia and genital warts. Both have possible long-term effects in females and may cause cancer of the cervix and pelvic inflammatory disease. The most recent STD is the viral infection human immunodeficiency virus (HIV), which attacks the immune system. Transmission is only possible by the direct exchange of body fluids and it is spread very easily during sexual intercourse.

The use of condoms, femidoms and dental dams are the only effective methods of reducing the risk of sexually transmitted disease as they form a barrier between body fluids. This reduces the chances of transmitting bacteria and viral infections. Although many STDs are treatable with antibiotic therapy, side-effects on psychological and physical health may cause long-term disorders.

3 Epidemiological and experimental evidence of disease and disorders

The study of the pattern of disease and disorders is known as epidemiology. Global, national and local centres have been established to investigate the distribution of specific diseases within a population, the aetiology of disease and the evaluation of the effectiveness of different types of treatment. Statistical evidence of morbidity (how many people are made ill by the disease) and mortality (how many people die as a result of the disease) is collected from health-care institutions and the registers of birth and deaths to provide information of social and biological factors relevant to disease.

The research methods used to study patterns of disease include the following.

Descriptive studies

Descriptive studies are based on data that has been obtained by routinely available information or surveys. This method is used to describe the pattern of disease. Using descriptive studies, social factors have been shown to clearly make a difference to health. The main factors are:

- Age.
- Gender.
- Marital status.
- Ethnic origins.
- Geography.
- Social class.

Analytical studies

An analytical study investigates relationships between health status and other variables. For example, descriptive studies may identify an increased incidence of lung cancer in men over the age of 60, analytical studies identify factors that are associated with the disease, e.g. smokers are more likely to have lung cancer. Analytical studies do not prove factors that are associated with the disease.

Experimental studies

If analytical studies indicate factors that may be associated with disease, experimental studies are then designed to prove an association between a given factor and the occurrence of the disease. Experimental studies may then provide information to prevent or treat disease.

There are many examples of successful experimental studies in epidemiology, for example spina bifida. Spina bifida is a congenital abnormality of the spinal cord causing a neural tube defect in which one or more vertebrae fail to develop completely. The defect may be a simple bony defect or it may involve a protrusion of the meninges or spinal cord. In severe cases there will be complete paralysis of the lower limbs. Descriptive studies showed that in the 1980s in the UK there was a 1 in 200 chance of a baby being born with spina bifida. Analytical studies identified that the percentage was higher in Northern Ireland than London, and it appeared that there was an increased rate in lower socio-economic groups. Many factors were taken into account including smoking, but after extensive analysis it appeared that diet was a possible cause. When analysing the dietary intake it was found that there was a possible link to folic acid intake. Experiments on a group of women showed evidence that the incidence of spina bifida was lower in those who had taken a folic acid supplement compared with those who had been given a placebo. Folic acid is now recommended for women a month before conception and during the first three months of pregnancy. The incidence of spina bifida has been greatly reduced in the UK.

The use of epidemiology in the area of public health provides information for health-service planning, health promotion, control of communicable diseases and evaluation and control of environmental hazards. Timmreck (1994) listed seven areas of epidemiology that benefit healthcare:

- History of disease: to show the trends of a disease for the prediction of trends. The results are useful in planning for health services and public health.

- Community diagnosis: identifying the diseases, conditions, injuries, disorders, disabilities or defects causing illness, health problems or death in communities or regions.

- Risks of individuals as they affect groups or populations: the risk factors, problems or behaviours that affect groups or populations. Groups are studied using risk-factor assessments and health appraisal approaches. This covers appropriate health screening, health risks etc.

- Assessment, evaluation and research: regarding how healthcare services meet the needs of groups and the population in terms of effectiveness, efficiency, quality, quantity and access relating to treating, controlling or preventing disease.

- Completing the clinical picture: identification and diagnostic procedures to establish that a condition exists and correct diagnosis is made. Determining the cause–effect relationship (e.g. identifying that a specific bacteria is the cause of a disease or disorder).

- The identification of syndromes: to establish and set the criteria that define syndromes. A syndrome is a group of signs and/or symptoms that when occurring together constitutes a particular disorder, for example Munchausen's syndrome.

- To determine the cause and source of disease: epidemiological findings allow control, prevention and elimination of the causes of disease, conditions, injury, disability or death.

Epidemiological studies have influenced government policies on all areas of healthcare. Coronary heart disease (CHD) was recognised as a major cause of death throughout the world and to investigate this disease the World Health Organization coordinated an international collaborative epidemiological study called Project MONICA (Multilateral Monitoring of Trends and Determinants in Cardiovascular Disease). The study took place over a 10-year period from 1984 to 1993 and the results published showed large variations in mortality rates for coronary heart disease throughout a number of countries and a great difference between the incidence in men and women. Mortality rates were far higher among people in lower socio-economic groups. All factors affecting coronary heart disease were noted, including links with age, gender, geography, smoking, high cholesterol and blood sugar (WHO, 1992). The results from measuring the trends in cardiovascular events have been used by many governments to plan health campaigns in an effort to reduce mortality rates. Statistics of the percentage of deaths in 1987, 1992 and 1996 show that circulatory disease is by far the main cause of death in England and Wales and the trend is increasing. In comparison, death caused by infectious and parasitic disease shows a marked decline.

In the UK the National Service Framework for Coronary Heart Disease (2000) was established for use within the NHS. The framework was set out covering seven areas in coronary heart disease management giving guidelines for practice to 'establish clear standards for prevention and treatment of CHD that will lead to major improvements in quality and access' (Department of Health, 2000). The areas chosen were aimed at reducing the incidence of heart disease, using health promotion campaigns to improve diet and reduce smoking, and improving immediate and consequent treatment.

Percentage of deaths by underlying cause which are certified by coroners with post-mortem examination, England and Wales, 1987, 1992 and 1996

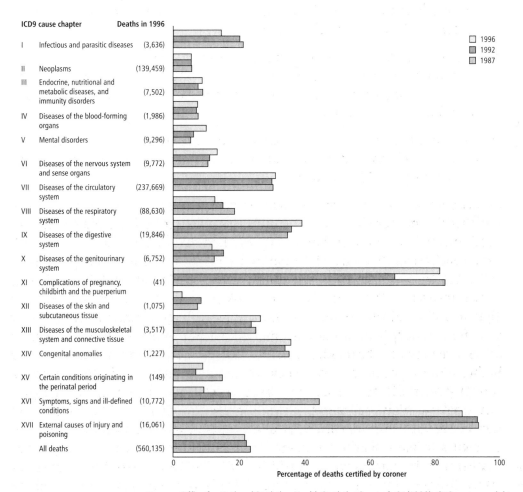

Source: Office for National Statistics, Health Statistics Quarterly 01(1999). © Crown copyright

4 The twenty-first century

The advances in knowledge and technology continue to expand rapidly, resulting in new and exciting changes in the area of healthcare.

Genetic work has not only identified causes of disease and disorders, it has opened a new field of science involved with human cloning and genetic modification and engineering. Stem cell research has shown that primordial cells may be cultured and potentially used to generate therapeutic tissue or spare organs. The therapeutic tissue might in future be used to regenerate damaged tissue and this may provide treatment for previously disabling conditions such as Parkinson's disease where stem cells are cultured to regenerate brain tissue. Burn victims would benefit from regeneration of damaged tissue by stem cells producing new skin tissue. Tissue engineering, using biodegradable synthetic materials, has enabled skin and cartilage to be grown in laboratories with further developments being made in bone, tendons, heart valves and intestines.

For conditions that require tissue transplant, human cloning may be seen as the first step towards the treatment of Human cloning has two distinct applications. The first is reproductive cloning in which a clonal embryo is implanted into the uterus producing a living child. The second application is therapeutic cloning that uses the cloning procedure to produce a clonal embryo that is then used to generate stem cells.

Human genetic engineering involves changing genes in a human cell. Somatic genetic engineering targets genes in specific cells. If a genetic defect is found, a viral vector (a virus-like organism containing new genetic material) carrying a healthy gene is inserted into the body. The viral vector attaches itself to the defective cell and is able to insert the healthy gene and theoretically the person will then be cured of the disorder.

Germline genetic engineering targets genes in eggs, sperm or embryos in the early stages of development. Alteration of genetic material affects all cells in the body and these changes will be passed on to future generations. Genetically engineered designer babies may be created by germline engineering using stem cell technology and embryo cloning.

Whilst the advances in genetic work give hope to those who suffer from presently incurable disease or disorders, the ethical implications of genetic engineering are immense and work in this field of science does not always meet with public approval. The Human Fertilisation and Embryological Act 1990 sets out stringent guidelines to prevent research on embryos past the fourteenth day of development. In the UK, licence must be obtained from the Human Fertilisation and Embryology Authority prior to research involving embryos. However, this does not prevent other countries from developing and introducing genetic engineering into healthcare. In communities that value male babies more than females, genetic research may be used to create the most 'desirable' baby.

Nanotechnology is another new science that it is hoped will lead to reduction of disease and disorders. Nanotechnology refers to the creation of engineered nanometre scale structures and their interaction with cellular and molecular components. By creating nanometre scale structures it is possible to control the fundamental characteristics of a material including, for example, changing its colour, magnetic properties or melting point without changing the chemical composition of the material. This has major implications for all industries including healthcare. A nanoscale device smaller than 20 nanometres will be able to easily enter the body's cells and transit out of blood vessels to interact with biomolecules on the surface of cells and within cells without causing any behavioural or biochemical changes. Nanoscale devices are able to hold tens of thousands of small molecules. The minute molecules inside the devices may hold any component including multicomponent diagnostic systems that are capable of assessing the metabolic state of cells or contrast agents that are detectable via magnetic resonance imaging (MRI). In cancer research it is hoped that 'nanotechnology will change the very foundations of cancer diagnosis, treatment and prevention' (National Cancer Institute, 2004)

The list of scientific advances occurring since the 1990s that have a direct or indirect benefit on health are too numerous to mention in this book. Each week new discoveries are made that will have an impact on global health. Unfortunately for us, nature is also creating new diseases and disorders that impact on health. MRSA, CJD and HIV are becoming increasingly common. On average, 13 people a day die in UK hospitals as a result of hospital-acquired infections (DOH, 2003) costing the NHS around £1 billion a year (DOH, 2003a).

Throughout the ages the effects that disease and disorder have on health have been linked to income and social class. In industrialised nations where healthcare is available to all, death rates have not changed as rapidly for the poor as for the rich. Poverty, unemployment, housing, diet and education are factors that must be taken into account when discussing mortality rates within a community. Although factors that affect disease are recognised, individual choice of lifestyle and habits are difficult to control or change. Coronary heart disease appears to be on the increase, although mortality rates have fallen (British Heart Foundation, 2003). However, it would be difficult to establish and then enforce a healthy lifestyle to be maintained by everyone.

Social, economic and political factors bear heavily on changing patterns of health. Technology, surgical procedures, drug therapy and healthcare enable many diseases to be cured, but often financial constraints limit the number of cases that are treated.

Geographical conditions are changing due to global warming. Diseases that were once seen only in hot tropical climates are now becoming more prevalent in Europe and the US. The ease of international air travel has increased the risk of epidemics and pandemics occurring. SARS, Ebola virus, Lassa fever, influenza and many other infectious diseases are transported quickly by the human vector from the original contact area to destinations throughout the world. Climatic changes will allow these diseases to thrive in previously hostile environments. The incidence of skin cancer in Caucasian populations is increasing at the rate of 3–7% a year and is now one of the most common cancers. HIV infection continues to thrive in all climates, bringing with it an increase in the incidence of tuberculosis, which in Africa is the leading cause of death in adults with HIV. Malaria carried by mosquito populations may become a hazard in the UK if infected mosquitoes escape from aircraft at British international airports and infect the local mosquito populations.

The quest for new improved drug therapies continues and research on vaccines and antibiotics for new and old diseases is assisted by the use of new technology.

There have been immense changes in healthcare and patterns of health throughout the centuries. This century must certainly be no exception with the promise of revealing answers to many of the mysteries surrounding disease and disorders. It is therefore interesting to note that alternative therapies, such as the use of larval (maggot) therapy (Sherman *et al.*, 2000), organically grown food and physical exercise, similar to the remedies recommended by many ancient civilisations are once again being advocated for use in modern healthcare.

Further reading

www.doh.gov.uk/publications.

References

Aylin, P., Dunnell, K. and Drever, F. (1999) Trends in mortality of young adults aged 15–44 in England and Wales. *Health Statistics Quarterly*, Spring edn.

Barnes-Svarney, P. (ed.) (1995) *The New York Public Library. Science Desk Reference*. Macmillan, US.

Black Report (1980) *Inequalities in Health*. Penguin, London.

British Heart Foundation (2003) *Coronary Heart Disease Statistics*. British Heart Foundation, London.

Department of Health (2000) *Modern Standards and Service Models*: *Coronary Heart Disease*. National Service Frameworks.

Department of Health (2003) *Getting Ahead of the Curve: A Strategy for Combating Infectious Disease*. Report from the Chief Medical Officer. The Stationery Office, London.

Department of Health (2003a) *Winning Ways: Working Together to Reduce Healthcare Associated Infection in England*. Report from the Chief Medical Officer. The Stationery Office, London.

Field, A. (2003) *Clinical Psychology*. Crucial Learning Matters Ltd, Exeter.

Government White Paper (1998) *Smoking Kills*. The Stationery Office Ltd, London.

Government White Paper (1999) *Saving Lives: Our Healthier Nation*. The Stationery Office Ltd, London.

Harding, S., Brown, J., Rosato, M. and Hattersley, L. (1999) Socio-economic differences in health: Illustrations from the Office for National Statistics Longitudinal Study. *Health Statistics Quarterly*, Spring edn.

Health and Safety Commission (1988) *Control of Substances Hazardous to Health Regulations 1988 – Approved Code of Practice*. HMSO, Norwich.

Myers, B. (2004) *Access to HE: The Natural Sciences*. Nelson Thornes, Cheltenham.

Prescott-Clarke, P. and Primatesta, P. (1998) Obesity in women: Higher levels among manual social classes. *Health Survey for England 1996*. The Stationery Office, London.

National Cancer Institue (2004) National Nanotechnology Initiative. www.nano.gov.

Office for National Statistics (1994) *Social Trends*. HMSO, London.

Priestley, J. (1905) Physical deterioration and alcoholism. Cited in the *Medical Annual 1906*, 556–557.

Sherman, R. A., Hall, M. J. and Thomas, S. (2000) Medicinal maggots: An ancient remedy for some contemporary afflictions. *Annual Review of Entomology*, **45**, 55–81.

Stranc, L. C., Evans, J. A. and Hamerton, J. L. (1997) Chorionic villus sampling and amniocentesis for prenatal diagnosis. *Lancet*, **349** (9053), 711–714.

Thomson, H. (2000) *Health and Social Care*, 3rd edn. Hodder and Stoughton, London.

Timmreck, T. C. (1994) *An Introduction to Epidemiology*. Jones & Bartlett, Boston.

United Nations Environmental Programmes (1989) *Environmental Data Report 1989/90*. Blackwell, Oxford.

World Health Organization (1992) *Our Planet, our Health: Report of the WHO Commission on Health and Environment*. WHO, Geneva.

World Health Organization (circa 1995) 'Death rates from circulatory disease: UK amongst highest in western Europe'. Health for ALL indicators database (EU), ICD-9, 390–459.

Abbreviations

Many abbreviations are used in healthcare. When using abbreviations, care must be taken that there is not more than one meaning (e.g. AA: Alcoholics Anonymous or the Automobile Association). The following list contains abbreviations that you may come across when researching aspects of anatomy and physiology relating to healthcare.

Ach Acetylcholine (as'-ē-til-KŌ-lēn): a neurotransmitter found at all nerve muscle junctions and other sites in the nervous system.

ACTH Adrenocorticotropic hormone (ad-rĕ'-nō-kor-ti-kō-r'-TRŌP-ik): produced by the anterior pituitary gland that stimulates the adrenal gland to release various corticosteroid hormones.

ADH Antidiuretic hormone: also called vasopressin, this is released from the posterior pituitary gland and acts on the kidney to increase reabsorption of water into the blood.

ADHD Attention deficit hyperactivity disorder: a behavioural disorder that is usually diagnosed when children reach the age of three to seven years.

ADP Adenosine diphosphate (ah-DEN-ō-sēn di-FOS-fāt): the chemical that takes up energy released during biochemical reactions to form ATP.

AIDS Acquired immunodeficiency syndrome: a disorder caused by the human immunodeficiency virus.

ANS Autonomic nervous system.

ARD Acute respiratory distress.

ARF Acute renal failure.

ATP Adenosine triphosphate (ah-DEN-ō-sēn tri-FOS-fāt): energy-carrying molecule that captures and stores energy.

AV Atrioventricular (a'-tre-o-ven-TRIK-yoo-lar).

BBB Blood brain barrier: specialised cells preventing passage of material from blood to the cerebrospinal fluid and brain.

BCG Vaccination: bacilli Calmette–Guérin: vaccination to protect against tuberculosis.

BMI Body mass index: an indicator of body weight, calculated by dividing the weight in kilometres by the height in metres. Normal range is 20–25.

BP Blood pressure: a measure of pressure in the arteries during ventricular systole and diasytole.

BPM Beats per minute: heartbeats per minute.

BS Blood sugar: the level of glucose in the blood.

BSE Bovine spongiform encephalopathy: a neurological disorder in cattle that is transmitted to humans causing Creutzfeldt-Jakob disease.

C Celcius: measure of temperature.

CABG Coronary artery bypass grafting: surgical procedure to bypass blocked coronary arteries.

CAD Coronary artery disease.

CCU Coronary/cardiac care unit.

CF Cardiac failure; cystic fibrosis.

CH Cholesterol (kō-LES-ter-ool′): a fatty substance and the most abundant steroid in body tissue, used for synthesis of steroid hormones and bile salts.

CHD Coronary heart disease: also called coronary artery disease.

CHF Congestive heart failure: inability of the heart to cope with workload.

CJD Creutzfeldt-Jakob disease: a rapidly progressive degenerative disorder of the brain.

CNS Central nervous system: consisting of the brain and spinal cord.

CO Cardiac output; carbon monoxide.

COAD Chronic obstructive airways disease: a disease in which there is some degree of obstruction of the airways.

CPR Cardiopulmonary resuscitation: administration of technique to restore life using external respiration and cardiac massage.

CSF Cerebrospinal fluid: fluid that circulates in the ventricles, central canal, subarachnoid space and the spinal canal.

CT scan Computerised axial tomographic scan.

CVD Cardiovascular disease: disorders of the heart, blood vessels and blood circulation.

CVS Chorionic villus sampling (kōr′-ē-ON-ik VIL-ī): a method of diagnosing genetic abnormalities in a fetus.

D&C Dilatation and curettage: a gynaecological procedure in which the cervix is dilated and the endometrium is scraped away.

DNA Deoxyribonucleic acid (dē-ok′-sē-ri′-bō-noo-KLĒ-ik): the principal molecule carrying genetic information.

DVT Deep vein thrombosis: a thrombosis or clot usually in a deep vein in a lower limb.

ECG Electrocardiogram (ē-lek′-tro-KAR-dē-o-gram): a method of recording the electrical activity of the heart muscle.

EEG Electroencephalogram (ē-lek′-trō-en-SEF-a-lō-gram′): a recording of electrical impulses from the brain.

ESR Erythrocyte sedimentation rate (e-RITH-rō-sit): the rate that red blood cells sink to the bottom of a test tube. Used to detect fibrinogen levels which are raised if inflammation or autoimmune disease are present.

F Fahrenheit: measure of temperature.

FAS Fetal alcohol syndrome: congenital defects that result from consumption of excess alcohol by the mother during pregnancy.

FSH Follicle-stimulating hormone: a gonadotrophin hormone, produced and secreted by the pituitary gland.

GAS General adaptation syndrome: model of stress.

GI Gastrointestinal: the digestive system consisting of the mouth, oesophagus, stomach and intestines.

Hb Haemoglobin (hē′-mō-GLŌbin): the oxygen-carrying pigment present in red blood cells.

hCG Human chorionic gonadotrophin (kō r'-ē-ON-ik gō-nad'-ō-TRŌ-pin): a hormone produced by the developing placenta.

HF Heart failure: inability of heart to cope with workload.

hGH Human growth hormone: hormone secreted by the anterior pituitary gland.

HPV Human papillomavirus: virus responsible for warts and genital warts.

HR Heart rate: the rate at which the heart contracts to pump blood around the body.

HRT Hormone replacement therapy: use of synthetic or natural hormones to treat a hormone deficiency.

HSV Herpes simplex virus: a common viral infection causing cold sores.

IBS Irritable bowel syndrome: a combination of abdominal pain with constipation and/or diarrhoea.

IUCD Intrauterine contraceptive device.

i.v. Intravenous: within a vein.

IVF In vitro fertilisation: a method to treat infertility by fertilising the ovum outside the body.

kPa Kilopascal: unit of pressure 1 kPa = 7.6 mmhg.

LH Luteinising hormone (LOO-tē-I-nī'-zing): a hormone secreted by the anterior pituitary gland.

MI Myocardial infarction (mī'-ō-KAR-dē-al in-FARK-shun): necrosis of myocardial tissue due to an interrupted blood supply.

mmHg Millimetres of mercury: unit of pressure.

MRI Magnetic resonance imaging: a scanning technique that produces a cross-sectional or 3D image of organs and body structures.

MRSA methicillin resistant staphylococcus aureus: a bacterium resistant to many antibiotic drugs including methicillin.

MS Multiple sclerosis.

MSU Midstream specimen of urine.

MV Minute ventilation: total volume of air inhaled and exhaled per minute.

NE Norepinephrine (nor'-ep-i-NEF-rin) also called noradrenaline: a hormone secreted by the adrenal medulla.

OD Overdose.

OT Oxytocin (ok'-sē-TŌ-sin): a hormone produced by the pituitary gland.

P Pressure.

PE Pulmonary embolism: blood clot or foreign body in a pulmonary arterial blood vessel that obstructs circulation to the lungs.

PG Prostaglandin (pros'-ta-GLAN-din): a fatty acid that contains hormone-like components found in all body cells except red cells; they act as a local hormone close to the site where they are released.

PID Pelvic inflammatory disease: bacterial infection of the uterus, fallopian tubes and/or ovaries.

PMS Premenstrual syndrome: physical and emotional stress occurring in the post-ovulatory phase of the menstrual cycle.

PNS Peripheral nervous system.

PRL Prolactin (prō-LAK-tin): a hormone secreted by the anterior pituitary gland.

PROG Progesterone (prō-JES-te-rōn): a female sex hormone.

PTH Parathyroid hormone: a hormone secreted by the parathyroid glands.

RBC Red blood cell; red blood count.

RDS Respiratory distress syndrome: a disease affecting newborn babies especially premature babies.

REM Rapid eye movement: the stage of sleep when dreaming occurs causing rapid eye movement beneath the eyelids.

Rh Rhesus: rhesus factor is the antigen on the surface of red blood cells.

RNA Ribonucleic acid (rī′-bō-noo-KLĒ-ik): used to decode DNA.

RR Respiratory rate: number of inhalations and exhalations taken during one minute.

SA Sinoatrial (sī′-n-Ātrē-al): the SA node normally initiates each heartbeat.

SARS Severe acute respiratory syndrome: a viral infection caused by the SARS associated corona virus (SARS-CoV).

SCD Sudden cardiac death.

SIDS Sudden infant death syndrome: the sudden, unexpected death of an infant without obvious cause.

STD Sexually transmitted disease.

SV Stroke volume: the volume of blood ejected by the ventricle in one systole.

SVC Superior vena cava.

T Temperature.

TB Tuberculosis.

TENS Transcutaneous electrical nerve stimulator: a method of pain relief using electrical impulses.

TIA Transient ischaemic attack: temporary interference of blood supply to the brain.

TLC Tender loving care.

TPR Temperature, pulse and respiration .

TSH Thyroid stimulating hormone: a hormone secreted by the anterior pituitary gland.

URI Upper respiratory infection.

UTI Urinary tract infection.

UV Ultraviolet.

VS Vital signs: heart rate, blood pressure, respiration and level of consciousness.

WBC White blood count; white blood cell.

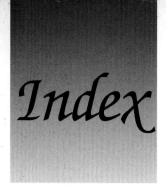

Index